Surgery
Mentor

Your Clerkship &
Shelf Exam Companion

SECOND
EDITION

Surgery

Mentor

Your Clerkship & Shelf Exam Companion

SECOND
EDITION

Robert A. Kozol, MD
Professor and Chair, Department of Surgery
University of Connecticut Health Center
Farmington, Connecticut

Yuri W. Novitsky, MD
Assistant Professor of Surgery
Chief, Laparoscopic Surgery
University of Connecticut Health Center
Farmington, Connecticut

F. A. Davis Company • Philadelphia

F. A. Davis Company
1915 Arch Street
Philadelphia, PA 19103
www.fadavis.com

Printed in the United States of America

Last digit indicates print number: 10 9 8 7 6 5 4 3 2 1

Acquisitions Editor: Andy McPhee
Developmental Editor: Andy Pellegrini
Manager of Content Development: George W. Lang
Manager of Art and Design: Carolyn O'Brien

As new scientific information becomes available through basic and clinical research, recommended treatments and drug therapies undergo changes. The author(s) and publisher have done everything possible to make this book accurate, up to date, and in accord with accepted standards at the time of publication. The author(s), editors, and publisher are not responsible for errors or omissions or for consequences from application of the book, and make no warranty, expressed or implied, in regard to the contents of the book. Any practice described in this book should be applied by the reader in accordance with professional standards of care used in regard to the unique circumstances that may apply in each situation. The reader is advised always to check product information (package inserts) for changes and new information regarding dose and contraindications before administering any drug. Caution is especially urged when using new or infrequently ordered drugs.

Library of Congress Cataloging-in-Publication Data
Kozol, Robert A.
  Surgery mentor : your clerkship & shelf exam companion / Robert A. Kozol, Yuri W. Novitsky.
—2nd ed.
       p. ; cm.
  Rev. ed. of: Surgical pearls / Robert A. Kozol . . . [et al.]. c1999.
  Includes bibliographical references and index.
  ISBN 978-0-8036-1695-0 (pbk. : alk. paper) 1. Surgery—Handbooks, manuals, etc.
I. Novitsky, Yuri W. II. Surgical pearls. III. Title.
  [DNLM: 1. Surgery—Handbooks. 2. Surgery—Outlines. WO 39 K88s 2009]
  RD37.S88 2009
  617'.9—dc22
                                                                          2008050045

To our Surgical Mentors

David Fromm and Demetrius Litwin

FOREWORD

The senior medical student and junior resident of today are faced with an enormous body of knowledge that they are expected to learn and utilize, often within short notice. Web-based information has gained a significant role in providing health-care providers with instant information. Studying, however, is still based in books. Like its predecessor *Surgical Pearls,* *Surgical Mentor* is a compact, succinct source of vital information for the student or trainee. It provides the foundation for solid surgical knowledge that is easily accessible. *Surgical Mentor* can be used during "down time" between OR cases and conferences. I believe that students and residents will find this small volume to be a valuable resource, easily tucked into their white coat pocket.

Walter Longo, MD
Professor of Surgery
Yale University School of Medicine

PREFACE

It has been 9 years since the publication of *Surgical Pearls,* and much has changed during the interval. Advances in minimally invasive surgery have allowed greater application of these techniques. The resolution of new-generation CT scanners and ultrasound has improved greatly. These improvements in imaging have altered the diagnostic approach to several abdominal conditions. The electronic medical record has improved efficiency for many practitioners. While technology has marched on, some things stay the same. For the medical student, the Surgery rotation remains a challenge. The student must still adapt to the "team approach" on Surgery and to the operating room culture. Senior students and junior residents are expected to accommodate a breadth of knowledge concerning a wide spectrum of diseases.

Surgery Mentor will serve as a rapid source of organized information in Surgery. Market research has revealed that today's student and resident prefer lists, outlines, and algorithms over prose. *Surgery Mentor* is therefore organized in outline form. Important facts are highlighted in each chapter, and each chapter is accompanied by practice questions. We believe that *Surgery Mentor* will prepare students and junior residents for conferences, rounds, and examinations.

Robert A. Kozol, MD
Yuri W. Novitsky, MD

CONTRIBUTORS

Heidi L. Fitzgerald, MD
University of Connecticut Health Center
Farmington, Connecticut
Chapter 3: Fluids and Electrolytes
Chapter 5: Minimally Invasive Surgery
Testbank questions and answers

Robert A. Kozol, MD
Professor and Chair, Department of Surgery
University of Connecticut Health Center
Farmington, Connecticut
Chapter 1: Introduction to the Surgical Service
Chapter 2: Instruments and Sutures
Chapter 11: Thyroid and Parathyroids
Chapter 12: Acute Abdomen and Appendicitis
Chapter 13: Stomach and Duodenum
Chapter 16: Pancreas
Chapter 20: Hernias

Tamar Lipof, MD
Resident Physician, Department of Surgery
University of Connecticut Health Center
Farmington, Connecticut
Chapter 6: Shock
Chapter 13: Stomach and Duodenum

Chapter 15: Spleen
Testbank questions and answers

James O. Menzoian, MD
Professor of Surgery and Co-Director
Collaborative Center for Clinical Care Improvement
University of Connecticut Health Center
Farmington, Connecticut
Chapter 21: Aneurysmal Disease
Chapter 22: Peripheral Vascular Occlusive Disease
Chapter 23: Cerebrovascular Disease

Yuri W. Novitsky, MD
Assistant Professor of Surgery and Chief of Laparoscopic Surgery
University of Connecticut Health Center
Farmington, Connecticut
Chapter 3: Fluids and Electrolytes
Chapter 5: Minimally Invasive Surgery
Chapter 6: Shock
Chapter 14: Hepatobiliary System
Chapter 15: Spleen
Chapter 17: Small Bowel
Chapter 18: Colon
Chapter 19: Anorectum

Brian Park, MD
Resident Physician
Department of Surgery
University of Connecticut Health Center
Farmington, Connecticut
Chapter 21: Aneurysmal Disease
Chapter 22: Peripheral Vascular Occlusive Disease
Chapter 23: Cerebrovascular Disease
Testbank questions and answers

Mun Jye Poi, MD

Resident Physician

Department of Surgery

University of Connecticut Health Center

Farmington, Connecticut

Chapter 4: Surgical Nutrition

Chapter 10: Breast

Chapter 14: Hepatobiliary System

Chapter 17: Small Bowel

Testbank questions and answers

Louis Reines, MD

Resident Physician

Department of Surgery

University of Connecticut Health Center

Farmington, Connecticut

Chapter 16: Pancreas

Chapter 18: Colon

Chapter 19: Anorectum

Chapter 20: Hernias

Testbank questions and answers

David Shapiro, MD

Resident Physician

Department of Surgery

University of Connecticut Health Center

Farmington, Connecticut

Chapter 4: Surgical Nutrition

Chapter 7: Trauma Evaluation and Resuscitation

Manish Tandon, MD
Assistant Professor of Surgery
University of Connecticut Health Center
Farmington, Connecticut
Chapter 4: Surgical Nutrition
Chapter 7: Trauma Evaluation and Resuscitation
Chapter 8: Burns

Steven D. Tennenberg, MD
Associate Professor of Surgery
Wayne State University School of Medicine
Assistant Chief, Department of Surgery and Director, SICU
John D. Dingell Detroit Veterans Affairs Medical Center
Detroit, Michigan
Chapter 9: Gastrointestinal Hemorrhage

Lori L. Wilson, MD
Assistant Professor
Department of Surgery
University of Connecticut Health Center
Farmington, Connecticut
Chapter 10: Breast

CONTENTS

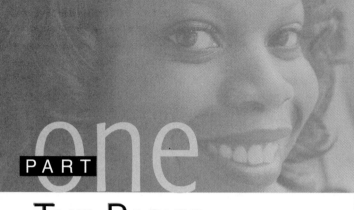

PART one

THE BASICS

INTRODUCTION TO THE SURGICAL SERVICE

Robert A. Kozol, MD

I. The Surgical Day

 Be affable, available, and enthusiastic.

A. Morning rounds
  1. Begin any time between 5:30 and 7:00 a.m.
  2. Team rounds versus individual physician rounds.
B. Work assignments
  1. Operating room (OR)
  2. Floor work
  3. Outpatient office or clinic
C. Late afternoon or evening rounds

II. Surgical Team

 Care of surgical inpatients requires teamwork. This includes close cooperation and coordination with all health-care providers.

A. Attending surgeons
B. Residents (chief down to juniors)
C. Students

Professionalism and respect for all lead to success and respect in return.

III. OR
  A. Personnel
    1. Nurses (may scrub or circulate)
    2. Scrub technicians (pass instruments)
    3. Anesthesia team
      a. Anesthesiologists (supervisor)
      b. Nurse anesthetists
      c. Residents
  B. Scrub technique
    1. Traditional liquid soap (scrub time 5 minutes)
      a. Unwrap brush and nail cleaner.
      b. Cover arms (to elbow) and hands with soap and water.
      c. Clean under fingernails.
      d. Use brush on each finger as if finger has four sides.
      e. Scrub palms and back of hands.
      f. Scrub forearms as if they had four sides.
      g. Rinse thoroughly.
    2. New rapid alcohol-based scrubs (scrub time 2 minutes)
      a. Apply to fingers, hands, and arms (to elbow).
      b. Reapply to fingers and hands.
      c. Rub into skin until dry.
    3. Scrub technician or nurse to gown and glove scrubbed team members
  C. Sterile fields

1. Most sterile areas are draped in blue or green; thus, a good rule is not to touch or brush against anything draped in blue or green.

 To avoid contaminating yourself once gowned and gloved, never touch your mask or drop your hands below your waist.

IV. Conduct of Operations
    A. Preparation

 If you know the operation to which you are assigned, read about it ahead of time.

        1. Positioning patient
        2. Team calls "time out" for correct patient, correct operation, correct body site (and/or side)
        3. Consider need for:
            a. Antibiotics
            b. Antiembolics
            c. Blood
        4. Hair removal (if needed)
        5. Place of lines and catheters
        6. Soap preparation (patient's skin preparation)
        7. Sterile draping
    B. Operation
        1. Incision

 When there are critical moments in the OR (uncontrolled bleeding, etc.), do not ask questions; wait until an appropriate moment.

        2. Exposure (retractors—see next chapter)
        3. Dissection and completion
        4. Closure
        5. Dressing application

V. Patient Recovery
    A. Time in postanesthesia care unit (PACU) or recovery room
    B. Transfer to floor or intensive care unit (ICU)

VI. Rounds
  A. Know your patients

  > If you scrub in on a case with a resident on your service, then you should see that patient postoperatively.

  1. History, physical examination
  2. Vital signs
  3. Laboratory test results
  4. Imaging results
  5. Fluids input and output
  6. Medication list
  7. Postoperative day (if applicable)

VII. Conferences
  A. Students may be bystanders or may be asked to participate (frequently asked to read radiographs)
  B. Reading radiographs
  1. Identify the film (e.g., "This is a CT scan of the abdomen.").
  2. Be calm.
  3. Be systematic.
     a. Bones
     b. Soft tissues
     c. Solid organs, etc.
  4. Do not jump to the obvious finding as you may miss something (again, be systematic).

VIII. Orders and Informed Consent
  A. Orders
  1. General
     a. Requirement for sets of new orders usually corresponds to events within hospitalization
        i. Admission orders
        ii. Preoperative orders—nothing by mouth (NPO) past midnight, preoperative antibiotics
        iii. Postoperative orders
        iv. Transfer orders
     b. Usually handwritten but increasingly electronic
     c. Best way to learn orders is to write them as a student, with appropriate supervision and co-signature

    d. To ensure completeness of orders

      i. Use mnemonics.

      ii. Visualize the patient from head to toe and cover all body systems.

   e. If orders handwritten, ensure legibility

   f. Always read over to yourself for accuracy before signing

 2. Generic order set mnemonic—ADC VAAN DIMIL

   a. Admit to _____ (service, attending)

   b. *D*iagnosis—i.e., S/P right hemicolectomy for colon cancer

   c. *C*ondition—i.e., stable, critical

   d. *V*itals—i.e., q shift, parameters for notifying resident

   e. *A*llergies

   f. *A*ctivity—i.e., bedrest, out of bed to chair

   g. *N*ursing orders—visualize the patient's nursing needs from head to toe

      i. Nasogastric (NG) tube to low continuous wall suction

      ii. Incentive spirometry (IS)

      iii. Jackson-Pratt (JP) drains to bulb suction, empty and record output q shift

      iv. Surgical dressing instructions

      v. Foley catheter to dependent drainage

      vi. Sequential compression devices (SCDs) to both legs

   h. *D*iet—i.e., NPO, clear liquids, regular

   i. *I*'s and O's—q shift

   j. *M*edications

      i. Antibiotics

      ii. Pain medications

      iii. Home medications

      iv. Other as needed

   k. *I*ntravenous (IV) fluids—e.g., D5 ½ NS with 20 mEq/L KCL at 100 cc/hr

   l. *L*aboratory test results

      i. Complete blood count (CBC), electrolytes in a.m. (date)

      ii. Chest x-ray (CXR)—specify portable or upright as needed

B. Informed consent

 1. General

   a. Required before performing any invasive procedure

      i. Surgical procedure in OR

ii. Bedside procedure—i.e., central venous line placement, thoracentesis

iii. Blood or blood product transfusions

b. Usually not required for minor procedures such as drawing blood, placing Foley catheter or NG tube

c. Must be obtained by physician; students do not obtain for medicolegal reasons

2. Specific procedure

a. Discuss procedure, reasons, alternatives, risks, and complications.

b. Offer patient to ask any questions.

c. Ask patients if they understand.

d. Document above on hospital-specific form as required.

e. Documentation usually requires a witness who will not be directly involved in the procedure—i.e., clinic personnel, nurse.

 MENTOR TIPS DIGEST

Be affable, available, and enthusiastic.

• Care of surgical inpatients requires teamwork. This includes close cooperation and coordination with all health-care providers.

• Professionalism and respect for all lead to success and respect in return.

• To avoid contaminating yourself once gowned and gloved, never touch your mask or drop your hands below your waist.

• If you know which operation to which you are assigned, read about it ahead of time.

• When there are critical moments in the OR (uncontrolled bleeding, etc.), do not ask questions; wait until an appropriate moment.

• If you scrub in on a case with a resident on your service, then you should see that patient postoperatively.

Chapter Self-Test Questions

Circle the correct answer. After you have responded to the questions, check your answers in Appendix A.

1. Describe four guidelines to follow when you are asked to interpret a radiograph.

1._____

2._____

3._____

4. _____

2. Give the key words for each letter in the generic mnemonic ADC VAAN DIMIL.

A _____

D _____

C _____

V _____

A _____

A _____

N _____

D _____

I _____

M _____

I _____

L _____

3. Give two guidelines to follow when writing orders to help you ensure you are not overlooking anything.

1. _____

2. _____

INSTRUMENTS AND SUTURES

Robert A. Kozol, MD

I. Overview

A. The most important tools of the surgeon are instruments and sutures. Although there are thousands of handheld instruments, familiarity with common instruments (Table 2.1) will suffice for the novice.

II. Scalpels (Fig. 2.1)

A. #10 blade (large incisions)

B. #15 blade (finer work)

III. Scissors (Fig. 2.2)

A. Metzenbaum (common for dissection)

B. Mayo (more sturdy for tougher tissue)

C. Suture scissors (cutting sutures)

TABLE 2.1	
Common Surgical Instruments	
Instrument Type	**Function**
Scalpel (knife)	Incisions and sharp dissection
Hemostat (clamp)	Grasping small blood vessels for hemostasis
Suture scissors	Cutting suture
Tissue scissors (many types)	Sharp dissection
Needle holder	Holding needle for suturing
Retractor	Moving body wall or organs to gain exposure

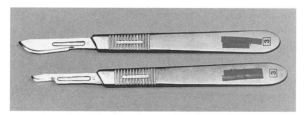

FIGURE 2.1 Scalpel with #10 blade, commonly used to open either chest or abdomen (*top*). Scalpel with #15 blade, used for finer work, such as excision of skin lesions (*bottom*).

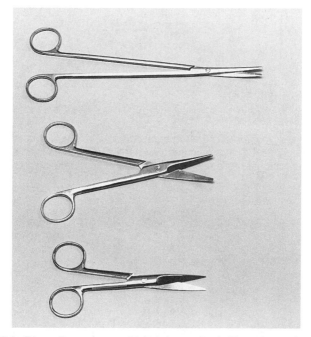

FIGURE 2.2 Dissecting scissors: Metzenbaum (*top*), Mayo (*center*), and straight suture (*bottom*).

IV. Forceps (Fig. 2.3)

A. Adson (skin)

B. DeBakey (delicate tissue and blood vessels)

C. Allis (ratcheted for holding sturdy tissue)

D. Babcock (ratcheted for holding delicate tissue such as intestine)

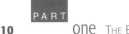

V. Clamps (Fig. 2.4)

    A. Mosquito (for small bleeders)
    B. Hemostat (for medium vessels)
    C. Kelly (for bulky tissue like mesentery)

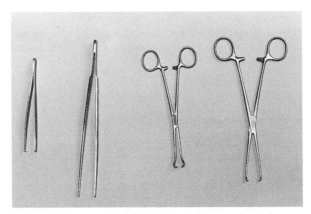

Figure 2.3 Surgical forceps: (*left to right*) Adson, used to pick up skin edges; straight tissue; Allis, used on tougher tissue such as fascia; and Babcock forceps. The Allis and Babcock forceps are sometimes referred to as clamps.

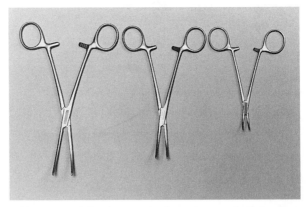

Figure 2.4 Hemostats (also known as clamps) come in three sizes: *(left to right)* Kelly, Crile, and mosquito, also called a snap.

VI. Retractors (Fig. 2.5)

A. Deaver (curved for organ retraction)
B. Body wall
C. Self-retaining retractor systems
   1. Bookwalter
   2. Omni
   3. Upper hand

VII. Sutures

A. Types
   1. Absorbable (Table 2.2)
   2. Nonabsorbable (Table 2.3)
B. Sizes
   1. The largest-diameter sutures have a single numerical digit for sizing.
     a. The largest (#5) is about the size of string.
     b. Zero (0) and #1 are commonly used to close fascia.
   2. Smaller sutures are followed by zeros (e.g., 2-0, 3-0, and 4-0). The higher the prefix digit, the smaller the suture.
     a. 9-0 and 10-0 are used for ophthalmologic and microvascular work.

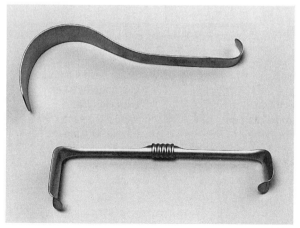

FIGURE 2.5 Deaver (C-shaped) retractor, which is often used to retract organs (intestine, liver, lung) (*top*); Richardson (L-shaped) body wall retractor (*bottom*).

TABLE 2.2 Common Absorbable Sutures			
Suture	Material	Duration of Tensile Strength	Common Uses
Chromic catgut	Submucosa of sheep's intestine	5 days	Internal gastrointestinal layer
Vicryl (Dexon similar)	Synthetic polygalactic acid (braided)	3 weeks	Internal layer of gastrointestinal anastomoses Small-vessel ligature Subcuticular skin
PDS	Synthetic monofilament polydioxanone	6 weeks	Fascial closure
Monocryl	Synthetic monofilament Polyglecaprone 25	2 weeks	Subcuticular skin

TABLE 2.3 Common Nonabsorbable Sutures	
Material	Common Use
Silk-braided	Small-vessel ligature Gut anastomoses
Nylon monofilament	Skin closure
Prolene monofilament (polypropylene)	Vascular anastomoses Fascial closure
Braided synthetic polyesters (e.g., Mersilene, Ethibond)	Fascial closure

    b. 3-0 and 4-0 are frequently used on the gastrointestinal tract.

    c. 4-0, 5-0, and 6-0 are often used for vascular anastomosis.

VIII. Laparoscopic Trocars
    A. Different sizes
    B. Cutting versus dilating

IX. Laparoscopic Instruments
    A. Designed to mimic conventional instruments
    B. Limited by design (long rods) with limited amounts of motion.

X. Hi-Tech Cutting and Coagulating Instruments
    A. LigaSure—bipolar clamp
    B. Harmonic scalpel—creates heat via vibration
    C. Lasers—many

FLUIDS AND ELECTROLYTES

Yuri W. Novitsky, MD, and Heidi L. Fitzgerald, MD

I. Anatomy of Fluid Compartments

A. 50%–70% of total body weight
B. Water content varies
  1. Body composition
    a. Proportional to skeletal muscle fraction
    b. Lower in obese people
  2. Age
    a. 80% of newborn weight is water
    b. 50%–60% of normal adult weight
    c. 40%–50% of elderly adult weight
  3. Sex
    a. Higher in males
C. Total body water (TBW)

 TBW is 60% of body weight, with two-thirds being ICF and one-third being ECF.

  1. Intracellular volume (ICV)—two-thirds of TBW
  2. Extracellular volume (ECV)—one-third of TBW
    a. Interstitial fluid (IF)—three-fourths of ECV
    b. Plasma—one-quarter of ECV or 5% of TBW

 Total blood volume is about 7% of body weight or, on average, 5 L in an adult.

      i. Venous side—85%
     ii. Arterial side—15%

II. Dynamics of Fluid Compartments

A. Hydrostatic pressure
  1. "Out" pressure
  2. Maintained by systemic blood pressure

B. Oncotic pressure
  1. "In" pressure
  2. Maintained due to impermeability of capillary walls to protein
  3. Albumin major determinant of capillary oncotic pressure

C. Maintenance of homeostasis
  1. Fluid shifts due to hydrostatic/oncotic pressures, electrolyte abnormalities, plasma osmolality changes
    a. Arterial and renal baroreceptors and atrial stretch receptors sense changes in effective circulating volume.
    b. Macula densa in kidneys senses sodium concentration shifts.
    c. Osmoreceptors in brain and liver sense shifts in plasma osmolality.
  2. Mediators
    a. Atrial natriuretic factor
    b. Adrenotrophic hormone
    c. Growth hormone
    d. Vasopressin
    e. Renin/angiotensin
    f. Epinephrine
    g. Beta-endorphins

III. Pathophysiology of Fluid Compartments

A. Global dehydration—decreased TBW
  1. Loss greater than intake
  2. Insensible loss (750–1000 mL daily)
    a. Water vapor from lungs, skin
  3. Sensible loss
    a. Stool (diarrhea)
    b. Urine (diuretics)
    c. Sweat (heat, exercise, fevers)
    d. Bodily fluids in drains

B. "Third space" compartment
   1. Pathologic space
      a. Fluid sequestered in tissue and cavities due to increased capillary permeability ("capillary leak")
   2. Stimulated by injury and/or inflammatory response
      a. Trauma
      b. Major surgery
      c. Intra-abdominal infection
   3. "Third-spacing" drains ECV
      a. Must be replaced even in case of increasing IF and TBW
      b. Crystalloid solutions preferred

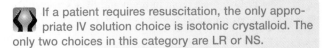 Two key fluids are normal saline (NS) and lactated Ringer (LR) solution. NS contains 154 mEq/L of Na^+ and Cl^-. LR contains 130 mEq/L of Na^+, 109 mEq/L of Cl^-, 28 mEq/L of lactate, and 3 mEq/L of Ca^{2+}.

If a patient requires resuscitation, the only appropriate IV solution choice is isotonic crystalloid. The only two choices in this category are LR or NS.

Dextrose is avoided for aggressive resuscitation because the body utilizes dextrose poorly in settings of severe stress, thus resulting in hyperglycemia. Hyperglycemia can cause an osmotic diuresis that will complicate the use of urine output as an accurate monitor of resuscitation.

   4. Failure to replace (and maintain) adequate fluid volume
      a. Decreased intravascular volume (plasma)
      b. Lowered effective arterial blood volume
      c. Systemic hypotension
      d. Decreased oxygen delivery
      e. Tissue ischemia and death

IV. Electrolyte Abnormalities
  A. Sodium (Na): overview
   1. Principal osmotically active particle
   2. Sodium balance linked to plasma volume

3. Regulation of plasma sodium occurs by changes in plasma osmolality

B. Hyponatremia (serum sodium <136 mEg/L)

1. Sodium deficit = TBW × (140 − [Na])
   a. TBW = 0.6 × weight (kg) for men; 0.5 × weight (kg) for women
2. Etiology
   a. Hypo-osmotic
      i. Hypovolemic
         (1) Gastrointestinal (GI) losses
         (2) Burns
         (3) Renal disease
         (4) Diuretics
      ii. Euvolemic
         (1) Polydipsia
         (2) Syndrome of inappropriate antidiuretic hormone secretion (SIADH)
         (3) Isotonic replacement of fluid losses
         (4) Decreased renal function
         (5) Adrenal (glucocorticoid) insufficiency
      iii. Hypervolemic
         (1) Renal failure
         (2) Cirrhosis
         (3) Cardiac failure
   b. Hyperosmotic
      i. Hypertonic infusion
      ii. Hyperglycemia
      iii. High concentration of glycerol, mannitol, glycine (transurethral resection of the prostate [TURP])
   c. Isosmotic
      i. Pseudohyponatremia (hyperlipidemia, hyperproteinemia)
3. Symptoms
   a. [Na] 120–130 mEq/L
      i. Apathy, confusion, lethargy, anorexia, nausea, muscle twitching, hyperactive tendon reflexes
   b. [Na] <120 mEq/L
      i. Convulsions, loss of reflexes, coma, death

4. Diagnosis
  a. Serum sodium
  b. Serum osmolarity
  c. Urine sodium
5. Treatment
  a. Identify cause
  b. Calculate sodium deficit
  c. Avoid rapid correction (central pontine myelinosis)
    i. 1.5 mEq/L/hr; 12 mEq/L/24 hr
  d. Water restriction in hypervolemia and euvolemia
  e. Isotonic saline in hypovolemia
  f. Hypertonic saline in extreme ([Na] < 110 mEq/L) cases or with severe symptoms
C. Hypernatremia
  1. Serum sodium concentration >146 mEq/L
  2. Hypo-osmolar state
    a. Free water deficit = 0.6 (TBW) $\times$ ([Na]/140 − 1)
  3. Etiology
    a. Hypovolemia
      i. GI losses
      ii. Sweating
      iii. Burns
      iv. Diuretics
      v. Glycosuria
      vi. Mannitol
      viii. Renal (acute renal failure [ARF], chronic renal failure [CRF])
    b. Isovolemia
      i. Diabetes insipidus (central or nephrogenic)
      ii. Hypodipsia
    c. Hypervolemia
      i. Iatrogenic
      ii. Cushing disease
  4. Symptoms
    a. Dry mucous membranes
    b. Neurologic symptoms
      i. Lethargy
      ii. Restlessness
      iii. Twitching

      iv. Ataxia

      v. Seizure

      vi. Delirium

      vii. Stroke

5. Treatment

  a. Identify cause

  b. Avoid rapid correction (cerebral edema)

    i. 0.5 mEq/L/hr; 12 mEq/L/24 hr

  c. Hypovolemia

    i. Hypotonic or isotonic fluids

  d. Isovolemia

    i. Free water administration

  e. Hypovolemia

    i. Free water and diuretics

D. Potassium (K) overview

  1. Major intracellular cation

  2. Normal homeostasis

  3. Physiologic serum concentration: 3.6–4.6 mEq/L

    a. 98% intracellular; 2% extracellular

      i. This [K] gradient affects resting cell membrane potential

  4. Regulation by kidneys

    a. Open potassium channels

    b. Na/K aldosterone-dependent pumps

E. Hyperkalemia (K >5.0 mEq/L)

  1. Etiology

    a. Impaired excretion

      i. Renal failure

      ii. Mineralocorticoid insufficiency

    b. Drugs

      i. Nonsteroidal anti-inflammatory drugs (NSAIDs)

      ii. K^+-sparing diuretics

      iii. Cyclosporine/tacrolimus

      iv. Angiotensin-converting enzyme (ACE) inhibitors

      v. Beta antagonists

      vi. Succinylcholine

    c. Pseudohyperkalemia

      i. Hemolysis

    d. Other

      i. Acidosis

      ii. Hypocalcemia

      iii. Insulin deficiency

      iv. Massive tissue destruction

      v. Compartment syndrome/rhabdomyolysis

      vi. Familial hyperkalemic periodic paralysis

      vii. Iatrogenic (excessive exogenous administration)

2. Clinical presentation

    a. Onset of symptoms with $[K^+] >5.5$ mEq/L

      i. Nausea/vomiting

      ii. Colic

      iii. Diarrhea

      iv. Electrocardiogram (ECG) changes

        (1) Peaked T waves

        (2) Widened QRS complex

        (3) Depressed ST segments

        (4) Loss of T waves (at higher potassium levels)

      v. Heart block

      vi. Diastolic cardiac arrest

3. Treatment

    a. Emergent with ECG changes

    b. Intravenous (IV) calcium (to stabilize myocardial membranes)

    c. Induce transcellular shift

      i. Glucose/insulin infusion

        (1) 50 mL of 50% glucose with 10 units IV insulin

      ii. Albuterol

      iii. Beta blockers

      iv. Sodium bicarbonate

    d. Promote total body loss of potassium

      i. Kayexalate15–30 g oral or rectally

      ii. Loop diuretics

      iii. Dialysis (in extreme cases or in renal failure)

F. Hypokalemia (K <3.0 mEq/L)

  1. Etiology

    a. Excessive loss from kidneys

      i. Diuresis

      ii. Mineralocorticoid excess

(1) Hyperaldosteronism
(2) Adrenal hyperplasia
(3) Cushing disease
iii. Renal tubular acidosis
b. GI losses (extracellular volume contraction with subsequent excessive renal potassium excretion)
i. Diarrhea
ii. Vomiting
c. Transcellular shifts
i. Beta agonists
ii. Inhalers
iii. Alkalosis
d. Inadequate intake
2. Clinical presentation
a. Ileus
b. Vomiting
c. Constipation
d. ECG changes
i. Low voltage
ii. Flattened T waves
iii. Depressed ST segments
iv. Widened QRS
e. Hyporeflexia
f. Cramps
g. Weakness
h. Lethargy, confusion
i. Paralysis
3. Treatment
a. Treat underlying cause
b. Avoid fast concentration changes
i. IV replacement
(1) Limit to 20 mEq/hr peripherally and 100 mEq/hr centrally
ii. Oral replacement
(1) Rapid onset—preferred method
c. Reverse hypomagnesemia
G. Calcium (Ca) and phosphate overview
1. Regulated by GI tract, bone, and kidney

2. Controlled by parathyroid hormone (PTH) from parathyroid glands
3. 98% of total body calcium and 99% of phosphate stored in bone and teeth
   a. Plasma calcium
      i. Ionized (50%)
         (1) Physiologically important form
         (2) Under tight hormonal control
      ii. Protein-bound (40%)
      iii. Complexed (10%)
H. Hypercalcemia
   1. Serum calcium >10.4 mg/dL
   2. Ionized calcium >1.25 mmol/L
   3. Etiology
      a. Primary hyperparathyroidism
         i. Parathyroid adenoma or hyperplasia
      b. Familial hypercalciuric hypercalcemia
      c. Malignancy (ectopic PTH)
      d. Vitamin D excess
      e. Hypophosphatemia
      f. High bone turnover
         i. Hyperthyroidism
         ii. Paget disease
         iii. Immobilization
      g. Thiazides
      h. Renal failure (secondary hyperparathyroidism)
      i. Milk-alkali syndrome
   4. Clinical presentation
      a. Musculoskeletal
         i. Weakness, fatigue
      b. Renal
         i. Diabetes insipidus (DI)/polydipsia
         ii. Acute and chronic renal failure
         iii. Nephrocalcinosis/nephrolithiasis
      c. Intestinal
      d. Anorexia, nausea, vomiting, constipation
      e. Neurologic
         i. Depression
         ii. Lethargy, confusion progressing to somnolence, stupor, coma

    f. Cardiovascular
      i. Short QT interval
      ii. Bradycardia and heart block
      iii. Arrhythmias
  5. Treatment
    a. Identify and treat underlying cause
      i. Aggressive hydration
      ii. Bisphosphonates
      iii. Calcitonin
      iv. Dialysis
I. Hypocalcemia
  1. Serum Ca <8.4 mg/dL
  2. Ionized Ca <1.0 mmol/L
  3. Etiology
    a. Hypoparathyroidism
    b. Hypophosphatemia
    c. Hypomagnesemia
    d. Chronic renal failure
    e. Vitamin D deficiency
    f. Liver disease
    g. Drugs
      i. Heparin
      ii. Glucagon
      iii. Protamine
    h. Infectious
      i. Toxins
      ii. Pancreatitis
      iii. Fistulas
    i. Pseudohypocalcemia
      i. Hypoalbuminemia
        (1) Measured calcium decreases by 0.8 mg/dL per
            1 g/dL decrease in albumin
        (2) Ionized calcium is normal
  4. Clinical presentation
    a. Numbness and tingling in circumoral area (Chvostek sign)
    b. Carpopedal spasm (Trousseau sign)
    c. Laryngeal spasm
    d. Mental status changes
    e. Convulsions
    f. Arrhythmias

5. Treatment
  a. Parenteral supplementation
    i. Calcium gluconate
    ii. Calcium chloride
    iii. Chronic calcium supplementation
    iv. Thiazide diuretics
J. Hyperphosphatemia
  1. Serum phosphorus >5 mg/dL
  2. Etiology
    a. ARF and CRF (uncommon with normal renal function)
    b. Exogenous sources
      i. Enemas, laxatives
      ii. Iatrogenic (total parenteral nutrition)
    c. Endogenous sources
      i. Rhabdomyolysis
      ii. Thyrotoxicosis
      iii. Growth hormone excess
      iv. Hypoparathyroidism
    d. Hypovolemia
  3. Clinical presentation
    a. Mostly asymptomatic
    b. Hypocalcemia leading to tetany
  4. Treatment
    a. Aggressive hydration
    b. Calcium carbonate
    c. Aluminum-based antacids (to bind phosphates in GI tract)
    d. Dialysis
K. Hypophosphatemia
  1. Serum phosphate <2.5 mg/dL
  2. Etiology
    a. Inadequate intake
      i. Poor diet
      ii. Diminished intestinal absorption
        (1) Vitamin D deficiency
        (2) Malabsorption
        (3) Diarrhea
    b. Excessive loss
      i. Diuretics
      ii. Burns

    iii. Liver resection/regeneration
    iv. Hyperparathyroidism
     v. Hyperaldosteronism
    vi. Renal tubular defects
  c. Cellular redistribution (from plasma to intracellular)
     i. Sepsis
    ii. Glucose infusion
    iii. Insulin
    iv. Glucocorticoids
     v. Epinephrine
    vi. Respiratory alkalosis
    vii. Leukemia/lymphoma
3. Clinical presentation
  a. Weakness
  b. Fatigue
  c. Rhabdomyolysis
  d. Cardiomyopathy
  e. Obtundation
  f. Respiratory failure
  g. Seizures
  h. Coma
4. Treatment
  a. Dairy products
  b. Oral phosphate salts
  c. Parenteral (IV) sodium or potassium phosphate
L. Magnesium (Mg) overview
  1. 50%–60% in bone
  2. Intracellular magnesium bound to ATP
    a. Essential to life
  3. Regulated by kidneys
  4. Excreted in feces and/or urine
M. Hypermagnesemia (serum magnesium [Mg] >2.9 mg/dL)
  1. Etiology
    a. Renal failure
    b. Acidosis
    c. Adrenal insufficiency
    d. Hypothyroidism
    e. Rhabdomyolysis
    f. Antacids

    g. Tissue injury, burns

    h. Severe extracellular volume depletion

    i. Familial benign hypocalciuric hypercalcemia

  2. Clinical presentation

    a. Toxicity exaggerated with concomitant hypocalcemia, hypokalemia, uremia

    b. GI manifestations

      i. Nausea

      ii. Vomiting

    c. Neuromuscular suppression

      i. Weakness, fatigue

      ii. Lethargy

      iii. Loss of deep tendon reflexes

      iv. Fascial paresthesias

      v. Hypoventilation

      vi. Paralysis

      vii. Coma

    d. Cardiovascular effects

      i. Peripheral vasodilation (cutaneous flushing)

      ii. Bradycardia

      iii. Hypotension

  3. Treatment

    a. Calcium gluconate

    b. Saline hydration

    c. Loop diuretics

    d. Dialysis

N. Hypomagnesemia (serum Mg <1.8 mg/dL)

  1. Etiology

    a. Diminished intake

      i. Poor diet

      ii. Iatrogenic

    b. Gastrointestinal

      i. Malabsorption

      ii. Fistulas

      iii. Pancreatitis

      iv. Diarrhea

    c. Increased renal losses

      i. Diuretics

      ii. Amphotericin B

      iii. SIADH

  d. Endocrine
    i. Hypoparathyroidism
    ii. Hypothyroidism
    iii. Hyperaldosteronism
    iv. Diabetic ketoacidosis
  e. Chronic alcoholism
2. Clinical presentation
  a. Toxicity potentiated by hypokalemia, hypocalcemia
  b. Gastrointestinal
    i. Anorexia
    ii. Nausea, vomiting
    iii. Dysphagia
  c. Neuromuscular
    i. Weakness
    ii. Paresthesias
    iii. Chvostek and Trousseau signs
    iv. Lethargy
    v. Confusion
    vi. Vertigo, ataxia
    vii. Tetany
    viii. Seizures
    ix. Psychosis, delirium
  d. Cardiovascular
    i. Arrhythmias
    ii. Ventricular fibrillation
    iii. Torsades de pointes
    iv. Cardiac arrest
3. Treatment
  a. Parenteral with magnesium sulfate
  b. Oral
    i. Milk of magnesium
    ii. Magnesium hydroxide

V. Volume and Composition of Gastrointestinal Secretions (Table 3.1)
  A. The deeper into GI tract, the more plasma-like secretions are in composition

 The deeper into the GI tract, the more plasma-like are the secretions in their composition.

TABLE 3.1	Composition of Gastrointestinal Secretions				
	Volume (mL/24 hr)	Na$^+$ (mEq/L)	K$^+$ (mEq/L)	Cl$^-$ (mEq/L)	HCO$_3^-$ (mEq/L) (mEq/L)
Salivary	1500	10	26	10	30
Stomach	1500	60	10	130	—
Duodenum	1000	140	5	80	—
Ileum	3000	140	5	104	30
Colon	—	60	30	40	—
Pancreas	500	140	5	75	115
Bile	500	145	5	100	35

Adapted from Shires GT, Canizaro PC: Fluid and electrolyte management of the surgical patient. In Sabiston DC Jr, (ed). Textbook of Surgery, 13th ed. Philadelphia, WB Saunders, 1986:74.

B. Secretions made in any GI tract segment absorbed in more distal portions of GI tract

C. Salivary secretions
  1. About 1500 mL/day
  2. Saliva relatively low in electrolytes, high in K$^+$ and HCO$_3^-$ content

D. Gastric secretions
  1. About 1500 mL/day
  2. Fluid rich in K$^+$, Cl$^-$, and H$^+$
  3. Patient with nasogastric (NG) tube or gastric outlet obstruction (with vomiting) may develop severe dehydration and hypokalemic, hypochloremic metabolic alkalosis

E. Ileum secretions

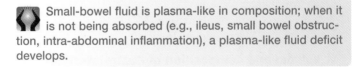

Small-bowel fluid is plasma-like in composition; when it is not being absorbed (e.g., ileus, small bowel obstruction, intra-abdominal inflammation), a plasma-like fluid deficit develops.

  1. Ileum mainly absorptive organ
  2. About 3000 mL of secretions per day
  3. Plasma-like fluid, normally absorbed by small bowel and colon

F. Pancreatic secretions

1. The pancreas secretes about 500 mL/day.
2. The fluid is very plasma-like, except for very high HCO_3^- (115 mEq/L).
3. In a patient whose pancreatic secretions do not enter the GI tract for subsequent absorption (e.g., pancreaticocutaneous fistula), IV fluids need to be supplemented with HCO_3^- to prevent a metabolic acidosis.

 The lactate in LR is rapidly metabolized to HCO_3^- by the liver, then converted to CO_2 in the blood and blown off by the lungs. It rarely affects pH.

G. Bile secretions

1. About 500 mL/day
2. Elevated HCO_3^- concentration (35 mEq/L)
3. Patient with excessive bile loss (T tube draining the common bile duct) likely to develop metabolic acidosis unless HCO_3^- supplementation given

MENTOR TIPS DIGEST

- TBW is 60% of body weight, with two-thirds being ICF and one-third being ECF.
- Total blood volume is 7% of body weight or, on average, 5 L in an adult.
- If a patient requires resuscitation, the only appropriate IV solution choice is isotonic crystalloid. The only two choices in this category are LR or NS.
- Two key fluids are normal saline (NS) and lactated Ringer's (LR) solution. NS contains 154 mEq/L of Na^+ and Cl^-. LR contains 130 mEq/L of Na^+, 109 mEq/L of Cl^-, 28 mEq/L of lactate, and 3 mEq/L of Ca^{2+}.
- Dextrose is avoided for aggressive resuscitation because the body utilized dextrose poorly in settings of severe stress, thus resulting in hyperglycemia. Hyperglycemia can cause an osmotic diuresis that will complicte the use of urine output as an accurate monitor of resuscitation.

- The deeper into the GI tract, the more plasma-like are the secretions in their composition.
- Small-bowel fluid is plasma-like in composition; when it is not being absorbed (e.g., ileus, small bowel obstruction, intra-abdominal inflammation), a plasma-like fluid deficit develops.
- The lactate in LR is rapidly metabolized to HCO_3^- by the liver, then converted to CO_2 in the blood and blown off by the lungs. It rarely affects pH.

Resources

Mont-Reid Handbook. Elsevier-Mosby, 2008.
Schwartz. Principles of surgery. McGraw-Hill, 2004.

Chapter Self-Test Questions

Circle the correct answer. After you have responded to the questions, check your answers in Appendix A.

1. Salivary secretions are typically about _____ mL per day.

2. Hyponatremia is defined as serum sodium less than _____ mEq/L.

3. Numbness and tingling in the circumoral area is a sign associated with which electrolyte imbalance?

4. Pancreatic secretions are very plasma-like except for very high _____.

See the testbank CD for more self-test questions.

4

SURGICAL NUTRITION

Manish Tandon, MD, Mun Jye Poi, MD, and David Shapiro, MD

I. Assessing Nutritional Status

    A. Anthropometric

> A subjective global assessment, consisting of a history and physical examination, is the best and simplest method of assessing a patient's nutritional status.

        1. Triceps skin-fold thickness
        2. Mid-arm circumference
    B. Clinical
        1. Recent weight loss
            a. 10% = mild malnutrition
            b. 30% = severe malnutrition
        2. Body mass index (BMI) = mass (kg)/height^2 (m) (Table 4.1)

TABLE 4.1	
BMI Interpretation	
BMI	**Description**
<15	Starvation
<17.5	Anoretic
<18.5	Underweight
18.5–25	Ideal weight
25–30	Overweight
31–40	Obese
>40	Morbidly obese

C. Laboratory
  1. Prealbumin
    a. Normal 16–40 mg/dL
    b. Half-life = 2–3 days
    c. Good index of short-term nutritional support
  2. Transferrin
    a. Normal 200–360 mg/dL
    b. Half-life = 8–10 days
  3. Albumin
    a. Normal 3.5–5.5 g/dL
    b. Half-life = 20 days
    c. Poor indicator of short-term nutritional support secondary to being an acute phase reactant and long half-life
    d. Low preoperative level strong predictor of surgical complications

II. Assessing Nutritional Requirements

A. 25–30 kcal/kg/day
  1. Protein 1 g/kg/day
B. Stressed patients require 35–40 kcal/kg/day
  1. Protein 1.5–2 g/kg/day
C. Nitrogen (N) balance
  1. Nitrogen balance = N intake − N output
    a. N intake—nutrition
      i. Amount of protein in grams per 24 hours divided by 6.25
    b. N output—urine urea, GI losses, open wounds
      i. 24-hour urine collection to measure urea nitrogen in g/day
  2. Negative nitrogen balance associated with malnutrition
D. Calculating daily nutritional requirements: Harris-Benedict equations

Caloric needs for average patients are 25–30 kcal/kg/day; protein needs are 1.0 g/kg/day. Preoperative nutritional support is of value in patients who have severe malnutrition (i.e., loss of more than 10% of body weight and an albumin level of less than 3).

1. Males = 66 + (13.7 × weight in kg) + (5 × height in cm) − (6.8 × age in yr)
2. Females = 65.6 + (9.6 × weight in kg) + (1.7 × height in cm) − (4.7 × age in yr)
3. Correction factors of basal metabolic requirement
   a. +15% for normal activity and work of breathing
   b. Additional stress factor corrections
      i. +10% in postoperative patients
      ii. +10%–30% in peritonitis
      iii. +30%–50% in trauma, sepsis, respiratory failure
      iv. +60%–110% in burns
      v. +5% for every degree Centigrade over normal in fever
4. Inadequate caloric intake
   a. Delayed wound healing
   b. Reduced ventilatory capacity
   c. Reduced immunity/increased risk of infection

III. Methods of Nutritional Support

A. Timing
   1. Preoperative support indicated in severe malnutrition or albumin <3 mg/dL

> Although albumin level has little value as a short-term index of nutrition during acute illness (long half-life of albumin is 21 days), a low (<2.8) preoperative albumin level does have a strong correlation with operative morbidity and mortality.

   2. Postoperative nutrition support indicated if diet not resumed in 7–10 days

> Elderly patients, with less nutritional reserve than younger patients, may require nutritional support by postoperative day 5 to 7, if diet has not resumed.

B. Enteral nutrition
   1. Use gastrointestinal tract if available, accessible

> Enteral nutrition is preferred over parenteral nutrition (if the gut works, use it).

2. Early enteral nutrition reduces postoperative mortality
   a. Prevents intestinal mucosal atrophy
   b. Supports gut-associated immunologic shield
   c. Attenuates hypermetabolic response to injury
3. Less expensive/fewer complications than parenteral nutrition
4. Forms of enteral nutrition
   a. Polymeric nutrition
      i. Short peptides
      ii. Medium-chain triglycerides and polysaccharides
      iii. Vitamins, trace elements
   b. Elemental alternatives
      i. L-amino acids, simple mono/disaccharides
5. Risks
   a. High osmolarity can lead to diarrhea
   b. Tube malposition or obstruction
   c. Gastroesophageal reflux and aspiration
6. Route: oral, nasoenteric, percutaneous/surgical feeding tubes
7. Method: initially low volume, diluted with gradual increases

C. Parenteral
1. Rationale: intestinal failure, usually secondary to reduced functional gut mucosa
2. Potential indications:
   a. Enterocutaneous fistulae
   b. Moderate or severe malnutrition
   c. Acute pancreatitis
   d. Abdominal sepsis
   e. Prolonged ileus
   f. Major trauma or burn injuries
   g. Severe inflammatory bowel disease
3. Peripheral parenteral nutrition
   a. Hyperosmolar solution
   b. Thrombophlebitis in peripheral administration
      i. Change catheter per appropriate schedule
   c. Limited nutritional supplementation
      i. 12 g nitrogen; 2000 kcal daily
4. Central total parenteral nutrition (TPN)
   a. Central venous access required
      i. Hyperosmolar, low pH: irritant to endothelium

b. Composition

> A standard TPN regimen is 20% dextrose (D_{20} with 5% amino acids at 80–100 mL/hr, with lipids given twice weekly. This provides about 2000 kcal/day.

  i. 14 g nitrogen as L-amino acids
  ii. Dextrose 15%–25% g
  iii. Lipid emulsion
  iv. Electrolytes
  v. Water-/lipid-soluble vitamins
  vi. Trace elements
  vii. Insulin
  viii. Acid suppression therapy
    (1) Proton-pump inhibitors
    (2) H_2-receptor antagonists
5. Parenteral nutrition administered via dedicated line

> Sudden unexplained hyperglycemia in a patient who had previously been tolerating TPN should alert one to the possibility of an infection, with line sepsis being high on the differential.

  a. Metabolic abnormalities develop in 5% of patients
  b. Excess or deficiency in sodium, potassium, or chloride
  c. Trace element and folate deficiencies
  d. Linoleic acid deficiency
  e. Hyperglycemia
    i. Insulin should be included in parenteral preparations to encompass half to two-thirds of a patient's daily insulin requirements, with correction scale or basal insulin provided separately.
D. Monitoring
  1. Clinically: weight stability
  2. Biochemically: Blood electrolytes twice weekly
  3. Nitrogen balance, magnesium, calcium, phosphate
  4. Liver function screening
  5. Weekly prealbumin and/or transferrin
  6. Line changed or replaced with any concern for line infection

MENTOR TIPS DIGEST

- A subjective global assessment, consisting of a history and physical examination, is the best and simplest method of assessing a patient's nutritional status.
- Caloric needs for average patients are 25–30 kcal/kg/day; protein needs are 1.0 g/kg/day. Preoperative nutritional support is of value in patients who have severe malnutrition (i.e., loss of more than 10% of body weight and an albumin level of less than 3).
- Although albumin level has little value as a short-term index of nutrition during acute illness (long half-life of albumin is 21 days), a low (<2.8) preoperative albumin level does have a strong correlation with operative morbidity and mortality.
- Elderly patients, with less nutritional reserve than younger patients, may require nutritional support by postoperative day 5 to 7 if diet has not resumed.
- Enteral nutrition is preferred over parenteral nutrition (if the gut works, use it).
- A standard TPN regimen is 20% dextrose (D_{20} with 5% amino acids at 80–100 mL/hr, with lipids given twice weekly. This provides about 2000 kcal/day.
- Sudden unexplained hyperglycemia in a patient who had previously been tolerating TPN should alert one to the possibility of an infection, with line sepsis being high on the differential.

Resources

Feldman M. Sleisenger and Fordtran's gastrointestinal and liver disease. WB Saunders, 2006.

Koretz RL. Do data support nutrition support?: Enteral artificial nutrition. Journal of the American Diet Association 107:1374–1380, 2007.

Owens C. Decisions to be made when initiating enteral nutrition. Gastrointestinal Endoscopy 17:687–702, 2007.

Chapter Self-Test Questions

Circle the correct answer. After you have responded to the questions, check your answers in Appendix A.

1. Write the Harris-Benedict equations.

  a. Males =

  b. Females =

2. Fill in the normal range of values for each:

  a. Prealbumin: _____ mg/dL

  b. Transferrin: _____ mg/dL

  c. Albumin: _____ g/dL

3. List a few reasons why if the gut works, you should use it.

  a. _____

  b. _____

  c. _____

See the testbank CD for more self-test questions.

5

MINIMALLY INVASIVE SURGERY

Heidi L. Fitzgerald, MD, and Yuri W. Novitsky, MD

I. Laparoscopic Surgery
   A. Minimally invasive surgery in the abdominal cavity
   B. Popularized in early 1990s
   1. Generally associated with decreased perioperative pain, decreased wound, improved cosmesis, decreased ileus, shorter hospital stay, decreased duration of convalescence compared with traditional surgery

    The major advantages of minimally invasive surgery are less post-procedure pain and shorter hospital stays. Pain is a major trigger to the neuroendocrine stress response to surgery.

   C. Abdominal cavity must be expanded during surgery
   1. Abdominal lift devices (uncommon)
   2. Pneumoperitoneum
      a. Insufflation of the abdominal cavity with CO_2

       The average volume of CO_2 required for initial pneumoperitoneum is 4 L.

      i. Preferred gas due to solubility and lack of flammability
      ii. Optimal/safe working intra-abdominal pressure: 10–14 mm Hg
      d. Intolerance of pneumoperitoneum may preclude a laparoscopic approach in some patients

II. Tools

A. Video equipment
  1. Light source
  2. Laparoscope (camera)
     a. Rigid tube with lenses
     b. Diameter 2–10 mm
     c. 0-, 30-, and 45-degree angles of the lens at the tip
  3. Video monitors
B. Gas insufflator

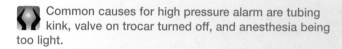

> Common causes for high pressure alarm are tubing
> kink, valve on trocar turned off, and anesthesia being
> too light.

  1. Warms and instills gas
  2. Monitors gas flow and intra-abdominal pressure
  3. Sounds alarm when pressure exceeds a set point
C. Trocars
  1. Cannulas (ports) for laparoscopic instruments/tools transabdominal insertion
  2. 2–12 mm in inner diameter
  3. Contain membranes for instrument insertion while maintaining air pressure inside
D. Laparoscopic instruments
  1. Graspers, dissectors, scissors, needle holders, biopsy forceps
E. Suction/irrigation
F. Laparoscopic energy sources for tissue division
  1. Hook electric cautery
  2. Ultrasonic (Harmonic) scalpel
  3. Electrosurgical bipolar vessel sealer (LigaSure)
G. Laparoscopic staplers
  1. Apply four to six rows of staples and divide the tissue in between upon firing, leaving two to three rows of staples on each side of the incision
  2. May be used for transection of viscera, mesentery, blood vessels
  3. May be used to create anastomosis (gastrojejunostomy, enteroenterostomy, etc.)

H. Hand-assist devices
 1. Allows placement of one hand in the peritoneal cavity while maintaining pneumoperitoneum
 2. Usually consists of a base ring placed intra-abdominally and a outer membrane creating a seal around the wrist/forearm
 3. Requires an incision 6–7 cm

III. Accessing an Abdominal Cavity
 A. Commonly done in the periumbilical area
 B. Proper technique crucial to avoid inadvertent injury
 C. May be particularly challenging in patients with previous abdominal surgeries (adhesions)
 D. Access techniques
   1. Veress needle—"blind" insertion
     a. Outer cannula with beveled needle point to cut through tissue
     b. Dull inner stylet that springs forward (clicks) on crossing various layers of abdominal wall and/or on entering abdominal cavity
     c. Protects underlying viscera from sharp tip of bevel
     d. When tip of needle in abdominal cavity, insufflator connected and position confirmed by low (2–4 mm Hg) pressure and/or saline injection
     e. On insufflation, trocar inserted blindly into abdominal cavity
   2. Open (cut-down) technique
     a. Fascia and peritoneum identified and incised under direct vision
     b. Stay sutures placed on fascial edges
     c. Blunt tip (Hasson) trocar inserted under direct vision
   3. Optical access trocars
     a. Combination of preceding methods
     b. Allows for laparoscope to be placed inside trocar to visualize layers of abdominal wall as they are traversed
     c. Requires experienced operator

IV. Physiology of Pneumoperitoneum
 A. Hemodynamic effects
   1. Decreased venous return (preload)
   2. Increased mean arterial pressure (afterload)

3. Decreased renal and visceral perfusion
4. Decreased stroke volume and cardiac output
5. Secondary tachycardia
6. Bradycardia due to excessive vagal stimulation
7. Compensatory changes may be affected by patient position
    a. Supine/Trendelenburg/reverse Trendelenburg
B. Effects of carbon dioxide (CO_2)
    1. Hypercarbia (usually transient)
    2. Myocardial suppression
    3. May induce arrhythmias
    4. Embolism (rare, given high solubility of carbon dioxide)
    5. Respiratory effects
        a. Decreased lung compliance (>30%)
        b. Decreased functional residual capacity
        c. Need for hyperventilation to excrete an increased carbon dioxide load

V. Risks of Laparoscopic Surgery
A. Pneumoperitoneum-related (0.7%–1%)
    1. Acidosis
    2. Arrhythmias
    3. Subcutaneous emphysema
    4. Pneumothorax
    5. Pneumomediastinum
    6. Atelectasis
    7. Gas embolism
B. Hemorrhage (0.6%–3%)
    1. Abdominal wall hemorrhage from trocar site
    2. Major vessel injury
C. Visceral injury
    1. Solid organ (spleen, liver) injury
    2. Bowel perforations during access or trocar placement (0.2%–0.3%)

VI. Pain After Laparoscopic Surgery
A. Visceral pain
    1. Predominant and most intense early
    2. Subsides after 24 hours
    3. Worsened by coughing but unaffected by mobilization

B. Parietal pain
   1. Lower intensity given small incisions
   2. Lasts 24–48 hours
C. Shoulder pain
   1. Neuropraxia of phrenic nerve
   2. Due to intra-operative diaphragm stretching/irritation
   3. Residual postoperative pneumoperitoneum
   4. Increases during first 24–48 hours
   5. May be only complaint
   6. May be minimized by lowered intraoperative pneumoperitoneum pressure

VII. Hand-Assisted Laparoscopic Surgery (HALS)
   A. Allows for a surgeon's hand to be inserted through a device (described earlier)
      1. Improves tactile feedback
      2. Facilitates organ manipulation
   B. Allows for an up-front use of an extraction incision
   C. Decreases learning curve of laparoscopic surgery
      1. Surgeon performance parallels open techniques
      2. Patient performance parallels pure laparoscopy
   D. Associated with clinical and immunologic advantages over open surgery

VIII. Clinical Applications of Laparoscopic Surgery
   A. Gastroesophageal surgery
      1. Laparoscopic esophageal (Heller) myotomy—proven benefits
      2. Laparoscopic Nissen fundoplication—proven benefits
      3. Laparoscopic gastrectomy—evolving
      4. Laparoscopic gastric bypass/banding—proven benefits
   B. Hepatobiliary surgery
      1. Laparoscopic cholecystectomy—proven benefits
      2. Laparoscopic liver surgery—evolving
         a. HALS usually performed
   C. Solid organ surgery
      1. Laparoscopic adrenalectomy—proven benefits
      2. Laparoscopic splenectomy—proven benefits
         a. HALS for very large spleen
      3. Laparoscopic nephrectomy—proven benefits
         a. HALS commonly performed

D. Colorectal surgery
   1. Laparoscopic appendectomy
   2. Laparoscopic segmental colectomy—proven benefits
      a. HALS often performed for sigmoidectomy
   3. Laparoscopic total colectomy
      a. HALS commonly performed
      b. Laparoscopic colostomy or colostomy take-down
E. Hernia surgery
   1. Laparoscopic ventral hernia repair
   2. Laparoscopic inguinal hernia repair
      a. Totally extraperitoneal (TEP) approach
      b. Transabdominal preperitoneal (TAPP) approach

MENTOR TIPS DIGEST

- The major advantages of minimally invasive surgery are less post-procedure pain and shorter hospital stays. Pain is a major trigger to the neuroendocrine stress response to surgery.
- The average volume of CO_2 required for initial pneumoperitoneum is 4 L.
- Common causes for high pressure alarm are tubing kink, valve on trocar turned off, and anesthesia being too light.

Resources

Assalia A, Gagner M, Schein M, eds. Controversies in laparoscopic surgery. Springer, 2005.

Jacobs M, Gagner M, Cueto-Garcia J, eds. Laparoscopic surgery. McGraw-Hill, 2003.

Chapter Self-Test Questions

Circle the correct answer. After you have responded to the questions, check your answers in Appendix A.

1. List two reasons why CO_2 is the preferred gas to expand the abdominal cavity for laparoscopic surgery.

   a. _____

   b. _____

2. List some of the physiologic effects of using CO_2.

_____

_____

_____

_____

_____

3. List some of the pneumoperitoneum-related risks of laparoscopic surgery.

_____

_____

_____

_____

_____

See the testbank CD for more self-test questions.

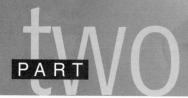

PART TWO

EMERGENCIES

6

SHOCK

Yuri W. Novitsky, MD, and Tamar Lipof, MD

I. Definition

A. Physiologic state marked by a significant systemic tissue hypoperfusion and resultant decrease in oxygen delivery.

 A shock state exists when there is inadequate tissue perfusion.

II. Pathophysiology

A. An initial (inciting) event induces a circulatory disturbance.

    1. Initial effects may be reversible

iii. Effects of Unrecognized/Untreated Shock

A. Cellular hypoxia

B. Derangement of critical biochemical processes

C. Breakdown of cellular membranes and intracellular components
1. Cell death
2. Organ damage
3. Multisystem organ failure
4. Death

IV. Physiologic Determinants of Shock
  A. Mean arterial pressure = systemic vascular resistance × cardiac output
  1. Systemic vascular resistance
      a. Determined by blood vessel length, blood viscosity, and vessel diameter
  2. Cardiac output
      a. Determined by heart rate and stroke volume
      b. Stroke volume depends on preload, myocardial contractility, and afterload (impedance to blood flow)

V. Stages of Shock
  A. Preshock
  1. Warm or compensated stage
  2. Adrenergic discharge
  3. Homeostatic mechanisms counteract initial insult
      a. Tachycardia, minor hypotension
      b. Peripheral vasoconstriction or vasodilation
  B. Shock
  1. Overwhelming of host regulatory mechanisms
      a. Tachycardia, tachypnea
      b. Hypotension
      c. Metabolic acidosis
      d. Cool (mottled) skin
      e. Oliguria
      f. Altered level of consciousness
  C. End-organ dysfunction
  1. Irreversible organ damage
      a. Renal failure (anuria)
      b. Obtundation and coma
      c. Systemic acidosis
      d. Multiple system organ failure
      e. Death

VI. Classification of Shock (Table 6.1)

A. Hypovolemic shock (decreased preload)

    1. Etiology

        a. Hemorrhage (trauma, gastrointestinal [GI] bleed, ruptured aneurysm) most common cause

        b. Fluid loss (dehydration, diarrhea, emesis, major burns, "third spacing": movement of body fluid into interstitial space) (Table 6.2)

TABLE 6.1

Classification of Shock

Type of Shock	System Dysfunction
Cardiogenic	Heart (pump)
Hypovolemic/hemorrhagic	Fluid volume (tank)
Septic	Infection/inflammation
Neurogenic	Arterial and venous tone

TABLE 6.2

Clinical Features Based on Severity of Blood Volume Loss

	Severity of Blood Volume Loss		
Clinical Features	Mild (<20%)	Moderate (20%–40%)	Severe (>40%)
Blood pressure	Normal	Normal	Hypotension
Heart rate	Normal	Slight tachycardia	Tachycardia
Respiratory rate	Normal	Tachypnea	Tachypnea
Skin changes	Pale and cool	Cool skin	Cold, clammy
Capillary refill	Normal	Decreased	Markedly decreased
Urinary output	Normal or slightly decreased	Decreased	Markedly decreased
Mental status changes	Unchanged	Restlessness, anxiety	Confusion, lethargy

. **B.** Cardiogenic shock (primary disturbance of the heart)
  1. Pump failure
    a. Decreased systolic function
    b. Decreased cardiac output
  2. Etiology
    a. Cardiomyopathies
      i. Myocardial infarction
      ii. Dilated cardiomyopathy
      iii. "Stunned" myocardium (post bypass surgery)
    b. Cardiac arrhythmias
      i. Atrial fibrillation or flutter
      ii. Ventricular fibrillation (may abolish cardiac output)
      iii. Bradyarrhythmias and heart block
    c. Mechanical abnormalities
      i. Valvular defects
        (1) Mitral regurgitation after ruptured papillary muscle or chordae tendineae
        (2) Aortic insufficiency after dissection of aorta
        (3) Aortic stenosis
      ii. Ventricular septal defects or rupture
      iii. Obstructing atrial myxoma
    d. Secondary (extracardiac) myocardial dysfunction
      i. Tension pneumothorax
      ii. Vena cava obstruction
      iii. Cardiac tamponade
      iv. Pulmonary embolus
  3. Clinical features
    a. Global hypoperfusion
      i. Systemic hypotension
      ii. Mottled extremities
      iii. Decreased urine output
      iv. Altered/depressed mental status
    b. Narrow pulse pressure
    c. Elevated jugular venous pressure
    d. Pulmonary edema
C. Vasodilatory shock
  1. Severe decrease in systemic vascular resistance, often with an increased cardiac output

2. Etiology
   a. Sepsis (most common)
   b. Systemic inflammatory response syndrome (SIRS)
      i. Widespread inflammatory response to a variety of severe clinical insults with the presence of two or more of the following:
         (1) Temperature >38°C or <36°C
         (2) Heart rate >90 beats/min
         (3) Respiratory rate >20 breaths/min or $Paco_2$ <32 mm Hg
         (4) White blood cell (WBC) >12,000 cells/mm³, <4000 cells/mm³, or >10% bands
   c. Toxic shock syndrome
   d. Anaphylaxis
   e. Addisonian crisis
   f. Neurogenic shock after severe brain or spinal cord injury

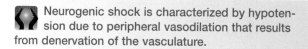 Neurogenic shock is characterized by hypotension due to peripheral vasodilation that results from denervation of the vasculature.

3. Clinical features

Septic shock is characterized by hypotension and a low systemic vascular resistance (due to vasodilatation and shunting), along with an increased cardiac output (hyperdynamic state) up to two to three times normal.

   a. Uncompensated (hypodynamic) stage
      i. Hypotension (not responsive to volume resuscitation)
      ii. Decreased circulatory volume
      iii. Third spacing
      iv. Tachycardia (bradycardia in neurogenic shock)
      v. Altered mental status
      vi. Oliguria/anuria
      vii. Cool skin, decreased capillary refill
      viii. Decreased central venous and wedge pressures
      ix. Decreased cardiac output (depressed myocardial function)

x. Peripheral blood pooling (altered venous capacitance)
xi. Widened arterial-venous (A-V) oxygen content
xii. Anaerobic metabolism with lactic academia
  b. Compensated (hyperdynamic) stage
    i. Increased cardiac output
    ii. Decreased peripheral oxygen utilization (narrow A-V O_2 content)
    iii. Normal or elevated central venous and wedge pressures
    iv. Hyperemic extremities
    v. Bounding pulses
    vi. Brisk capillary refill
    vii. Wide pulse pressure

VII. History, Physical Examination, Laboratory Test Results, and Imaging

  A. History
    1. Patient may not be able to provide information
    2. Data garnered form relatives, friends, caretakers, or medical records
    3. General condition
    4. Recent events (accidents, exposures, travel)
    5. Recent complaints
    6. Activities before presentation
  B. Physical examination—directed to establish the diagnosis, uncover underlying cause
    1. Primary survey
      a. Assessment and establishment of an airway
      b. Evaluation for mechanical ventilation
      c. Restoration of circulatory volume
    2. Secondary survey
      a. Varies with presentation, cause of shock, stage of resuscitation
      b. Head, ears, eyes, nose, and throat (HEENT): pupils, mucous membranes
      c. CHEST: tachypnea, labored breathing, rales, absent breath sounds
      d. Cardiovascular (CV): arrhythmias, murmurs, distant heart sounds

    e. GI: abdominal distention, tenderness, masses, acute or occult bleeding, decreased rectal tone

    f. SKIN: cold or warm, clammy, mottled, rash, cellulitis, urticaria

    g. NEUROLOGIC: agitation, confusion, delirium, obtundation, coma, reflexes

C. Laboratory evaluation

    1. Blood

        a. Complete blood count

        b. Basic and liver chemistries

        c. Amylase and lipase

        d. Lactate

        e. Cardiac enzymes

        f. Arterial blood gases

        g. Toxicology

    2. Urine

        a. Urinalysis

        b. Urine osmolarity, creatinine, sodium

        c. Calculation of fractional secretion of sodium (FENA)

    3. Microbiology

        a. Blood cultures

        b. Urine cultures

D. Imaging

    1. Chest radiograph

    2. Abdominal radiograph (obstructive series)

    3. Extremity radiographs

    4. Computed tomography

VIII. Treatment of Shock (Table 6.3)

 The management of shock begins with the ABCs of life support.

A. Endpoints of resuscitation

    1. Mean arterial pressure: 60–65 mm Hg

    2. Central venous pressure (CVP): 8–12 cm H_2O

    3. Urine output >0.5 mL/kg/hr

    4. Mixed venous oxygen saturation >70%

    5. Normal lactate and based deficit

    6. Control of hyperglycemia (glucose 80–110 mg/dL)

TABLE 6.3
General Treatment of Shock States

Type of Shock	Treatment
Cardiogenic	
Myocardial infarction	Coronary vasodilators
	Diuresis (preload and afterload reduction)
Cardiac tamponade	Pericardiocentesis, pericardial window
	Surgery to correct underlying cardiac injury
Hypovolemic	Isotonic crystalloid resuscitation
Hemorrhagic	Isotonic crystalloid resuscitation
	Blood if loss ≥30% total blood volume
Septic	Isotonic crystalloid resuscitation
	Surgery to drain pus or resolve perforation
	Antibiotics
Neurogenic	Isotonic crystalloid resuscitation

B. Hemorrhagic shock
   1. Identify and control the hemorrhage.
   2. Restore circulating volume.

 The initial management of hypovolemic shock is prompt and requires aggressive fluid resuscitation.

   a. Crystalloid volume three times the blood loss (3-to-1 rule)

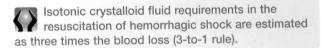 Isotonic crystalloid fluid requirements in the resuscitation of hemorrhagic shock are estimated as three times the blood loss (3-to-1 rule).

   b. Blood products
   c. Must be done during/after a definitive intervention to stop hemorrhage
   3. Restore oxygen perfusion to the tissues.
   4. Avoid vasopressors.
C. Cardiogenic shock
   1. Establish etiology
   2. Fluid resuscitation (unless congestive heart failure [CHF])

3. Stress-ulcer prophylaxis
4. Vasoactive therapy
   a. Dobutamine
   b. Dopamine
   c. Neo-Synephrine
   d. Amrinone
5. Intra-aortic balloon pump
6. Revascularization in the setting of acute myocardial infarction (MI)
   a. Anti-platelet agents
   b. Systemic anticoagulation
   c. Thrombolytics
   d. Angioplasty
   e. Cardiac (bypass, valve repair) surgery
D. Septic shock
   1. Fluid resuscitation

 Aggressive and rapid volume resuscitation must always precede surgical intervention for septic shock.

   2. Control of infection
      a. Empiric broad-spectrum antibiotics
      b. Abscess drainage
      c. Surgical débridement
   3. Vasopressor therapy (Table 6.4)
      a. Levophed
      b. Neo-Synephrine
      c. Vasopressin
      d. Dopamine (falling out of favor)
   4. Stress-ulcer prophylaxis
   5. Aggressive blood glucose control (improves survival)
   6. Recombinant human-activated protein C (Zyvox) and low-dose corticosteroids
      a. Decreases mortality based on prospective randomized trials

 Infections are the leading cause of death after management of shock.

TABLE 6.4

Common Cardiovascular Agents

Agent	Dose range (mcg/kg/min)	Other Major Effects
Inotropes		
Dopamine	2–15	Renal/mesenteric vasodilation at low doses
Dobutamine	2–15	Vasodilation
Amrinone	5–15	Vasodilation
Vasopressors		
Norepinephrine	0.05–0.2	Inotrope
Epinephrine	0.03–0.2	Inotrope/chronotrope at low doses
Phenylephrine	0.6–2	Pure alpha vasoconstrictor
Vasodilators		
Nitroglycerin	0.2–2	Coronary vasodilation
Nitroprusside	1–5	Pure vasodilator

MENTOR TIPS DIGEST

- A shock state exists when there is inadequate tissue perfusion.
- Neurogenic shock is characterized by hypotension due to peripheral vasodilation that results from denervation of the vasculature.
- Septic shock is characterized by hypotension and a low systemic vascular resistance (due to vasodilatation and shunting), along with an increased cardiac output (hyperdynamic state) up to two to three times normal.
- The management of shock begins with the ABCs of life support.
- The initial management of hypovolemic shock is prompt and requires aggressive fluid resuscitation.
- Isotonic crystalloid fluid requirements in the resuscitation of hemorrhagic shock are estimated as three times the blood loss (3-to-1 rule).
- Aggressive and rapid volume resuscitation must always precede surgical intervention for septic shock.
- Infections are the leading cause of death after management of shock.

Resources

Cunha BA. Sepsis and septic shock: Selection of empiric antimicrobial therapy. Critical Care Clinics 24:313–334, 2008.

Fink MP. Textbook of critical care, 5th ed. Elsevier, 2005.

Chapter Self-Test Questions

Circle the correct answer. After you have responded to the questions, check your answers in Appendix A.

1. The approximate mean arterial pressure is calculated by multiplying:

    a. Heart rate (HR) × stroke volume (SV)

    b. Cardiac output (CO)/body surface area (BSA)

    c. Stroke volume (SV)/body surface area (BSA)

    d. Systemic vascular resistance (SVR) × cardiac output (CO)

2. All of the following are systemic inflammatory response syndrome (SIRS) criteria *except:*

    a. HR >90 bpm

    b. Temperature <36°C or >38°C

    c. Bacteremia

    d. Respiratory rate (RR) >20 or $Paco_2$ <32 mm Hg

    e. WBC <4000 or >12,000 or 10% bands

3. Shock state is best characterized by:

    a. Hypotension

    b. Inadequate tissue perfusion

    c. Tachycardia

    d. Acidosis

4. Isotonic crystalloid fluid requirements in the resuscitation of hemorrhagic shock are administered at a rate approximately how many times the blood loss:

   a. 1:1

   b. 2:1

   c. 3:1

   d. 4:1

5. Causes of cardiogenic shock include all of the following *except:*

   a. Acute myocardial infarction

   b. Cardiac tamponade

   c. Aortic stenosis

   d. Pneumonia

   e. Malignant hypertension

 See the testbank CD for more self-test questions.

7

TRAUMA EVALUATION AND RESUSCITATION

Manish Tandon, MD, and David Shapiro, MD

I. Trauma Overview
A. Extent of problem
  1. 2 million hospitalizations and more than 160,000 deaths per year
  2. Fifth leading cause of death overall; leading cause of death for ages 1–44 years
  3. Costs more than $100 billion per year in medical costs
B. What it includes
  1. Leading causes of injury-related deaths
    a. Motor vehicle crashes
    b. Suicide
    c. Homicide
    d. Drowning
    e. Fires
  2. Risks exist at any age
    a. Younger than 1 year old—unintentional suffocation, child maltreatment
    b. Years 1–4: motor vehicle crashes (unrestrained), drowning, child maltreatment
    c. Years 4–11: motor vehicle crashes (no booster seat), drowning, homicide (firearms)
    d. Years 12–19: motor vehicle crashes (unbelted, intoxicated), homicide, suicide, sports injuries
    e. Years 20–49: motor vehicle crashes, homicide, suicide, falls
    f. Years 50 and older: falls, motor vehicle crashes, suicide

C. Trauma centers
   1. Designated by states, often verified by American College of Surgeons
   2. Level I—full trauma capabilities, including research and outreach
   3. Level II—full trauma capabilities
   4. Level III—continuous general surgery and orthopedics coverage
   5. Level IV—Initial evaluation and assessment
D. Scoring systems
   1. Used to predict mortality, to identify unexpected deaths
   2. Injury severity score (ISS)—to predict mortality
      a. Sum of the squares of the three highest abbreviated injury scale (AIS) scores (each 1–5)
   3. Trauma injury severity score (TRISS)—combination of ISS and revised trauma score (RTS)
E. Prevention
   1. Fall prevention for elderly
   2. Fire safety with smoke alarms
   3. Booster seats, seat belts, air bags, car design
   4. Interventions for alcohol-impaired driving
   5. Violence prevention programs
F. Shock (see Chapter 6)

II. Assessment of Trauma Patient
A. Primary survey *(ABCDE)*
   1. *A*irway
      a. Patency of airway assessed

> The quickest way of ensuring a patent, working airway, as well as a conscious, mentally alert patient, is by getting an appropriate verbal response after asking a patient how he or she is doing.

      i. Visual and verbal assessments
      ii. Maxillofacial or laryngeal trauma
   b. Jaw thrust or chin lift

> In trauma, all patients are considered to have a cervical spinal cord injury and are treated accordingly until it has been proved.that no such injury exists. Maintain neck immobilization throughout initial management.

> If the chin lift and jaw thrust fail to establish a patent airway or if the patient is unresponsive, advanced airway intervention with oral endotracheal or nasotracheal intubation is required.

    c. Oral airway if no gag reflex
    d. Bag-valve mask ventilation
    e. Rapid sequence intubation
        i. Preoxygenate
        ii. C-spine stabilization
        iii. Cricoid pressure
        iv. Fast- and short-acting paralytic such as succinylcholine
        v. Possible use of lidocaine and/or induction agent such as etomidate
        vi. Oral endotracheal tube placement
        vii. Confirm breath sounds and $ETCO_2$ before releasing cricoid pressure
    f. Surgical airway
    g. Maintain C-spine precautions throughout all preceding
2. *B*reathing

> Three life-threatening ventilatory conditions that must be recognized and treated in the primary survey are tension pneumothorax, open pneumothorax, and flail chest with pulmonary contusion.

    a. Assess for bilateral breath sounds and pulse oximetry.
    b. Adjust endotracheal tube (ETT) position if needed.
    c. Check pneumothorax or hemothorax.
        i. Needle decompression if unstable
        ii. Chest tube for definitive treatment

3. *C*irculation
   a. Assess manual blood pressure, central and peripheral pulses

   > During the primary survey, circulation is assessed by checking three parameters: mental status, skin color, and hemodynamic status (heart rate and blood pressure).

   b. Establish intravenous (IV) access—peripheral, central, intraosseus; draw blood sample
   c. Hypotension

   > Hemodynamic instability, defined as heart rate (HR) greater than 100 or systolic blood pressure less than 90, is considered due to blood loss until proved otherwise.

   > The classic triad (Beck triad) of hypotension, distended neck veins, and muffled heart sounds is present in fewer than half of patients who are found to have pericardial tamponade.

      i. Warm crystalloid
        (1) 1–2 L bolus for adults
        (2) 20 mL/kg for pediatrics
     ii. Blood
        (1) If no response to 2 L or 2–3 boluses of 20 mL/kg
        (2) Uncross-matched blood
        (3) O negative if female of childbearing age
        (4) 10 mL/kg packed red blood cells (PRBCs) in pediatrics

   > The resuscitation phase consists of providing supplemental oxygen, beginning fluid resuscitation with 2 L lactated Ringer solution via two large-bore peripheral IV lines, ECG monitoring, nasogastric tube and Foley insertion, and laboratory evaluation.

iii. Sources of hemorrhage
(1) Intrathoracic—chest x-ray (CXR) or chest tubes
(2) Intra-abdominal—focused assessment by sonography for trauma (FAST) or diagnostic peritoneal lavage (DPL); computed tomography (CT) scan if stabilized
(3) Retroperitoneal—pelvis x-ray; CT scan when stabilized
(4) Long bones
(5) External—lacerations, scalp lacerations, open fractures
iv. Patient kept warm
4. *D*isability
   a. Assess consciousness
      i. Alert
      ii. Verbal—responds to verbal stimuli
      iii. Pain—responds to painful stimuli
      iv. Unresponsive to all stimuli
   b. Assess for movement in all extremities
5. *E*xposure
   a. Remove all clothing to assess for wounds, deformities
   b. Check temperature for and prevent hypothermia
   c. Cover patient with warm, dry blankets
6. Simultaneous assessment and history and resuscitation if unstable
7. Electrocardiogram (ECG) monitoring, possible gastric and urinary catheters
   a. No nasal tubes if any concern for mid-face fractures
   b. Contraindications to placing urinary catheter before retrograde urethrogram
      i. Blood at penile meatus
      ii. High-riding prostate
      iii. Scrotal hematoma
B. Secondary survey and immediate tests
   1. Potential emergency department tests
      a. C-spine, CXR, pelvis x-ray, FAST

 Three x-rays are mandatory in all trauma patients: lateral cervical spine, chest, and pelvis.

b. Before or after secondary survey depending on stability
2. History *(AMPLE)*
   a. *A*llergies
   b. *M*edications
   c. *P*ast illnesses/*P*regnancy
   d. *L*ast meal
   e. *E*vents/*E*nvironment
      i. Patterns of injury (e.g., pedestrian struck by motor vehicle or frontal impact)
3. Secondary survey head-to-toe examination
   a. Assess all areas for tenderness, deformities, wounds, bleeding, passive and active range of motion
   b. Head, including papillary reaction, ear canal drainage
   c. Neurologic examination
      i. Assess Glasgow Coma Scale (GCS)
         (1) Eye (E)
            (A) Spontaneous—4 points
            (B) To verbal stimuli—3 points
            (C) To painful stimuli—2 points
            (D) No eye opening—1 point
         (2) Verbal (V)
            (A) Oriented—5 points
            (B) Confused—4 points
            (C) Inappropriate words—3 points
            (D) Incomprehensible sounds—2 points
            (E) No sound or intubated—1 point
         (3) Motor (M)
            (A) Follows commands—6 points
            (B) Localizes to pain—5 points
            (C) Withdraws to pain—4 points
            (D) Abnormal flexion/decorticate posturing—3 points
            (E) Abnormal extension/decerebrate posturing—2 points
            (F) No movement, flaccid—1 point
      ii. GCS score is 8 or less than 8, patient will need airway secured
   d. Facial bones
      i. Reassess aspiration of blood
      ii. Malocclusion

e. Neck/C-spine
  i. Assume C-spine injury; maintain spine precautions.
  ii. Reassess for tracheal deviation, laryngeal tenderness, crepitus, bruits, hematomas, hoarseness, dysphagia
  iii. Penetrating injuries to neck
    (1) Zone I
      (A) Clavicles to cricoid cartilage
    (2) Zone II
      (A) Cricoid cartilage to angle of mandible
    (3) Zone III
      (A) Above angle of mandible
f. Chest
  i. Reassess breath sounds, heart sounds; check for crepitus
  ii. Stab wound to chest
    (1) Chest tube if decreased breath sounds, hypoxia, sucking chest wound
    (2) If no pneumothorax (PTX) on initial x-ray, repeat x-ray in 6–8 hours
  iii. Stab wound to "box" ("box" is part of anterior chest and abdomen; bounded by clavicles superiorly, midclavicular lines laterally, and costal margin in midclavicular line.)
    (1) Midclavicular lines, from nipples to costal margin
    (2) High suspicion for cardiac injury
    (3) FAST for initial screening
    (4) Formal ultrasound (if no fluid on FAST) and stable
    (5) Pericardial window or operative repair if positive FAST for pericardial fluid

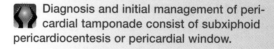

Diagnosis and initial management of pericardial tamponade consist of subxiphoid pericardiocentesis or pericardial window.

g. Abdomen
  i. Tenderness
    (1) Worsening or persistent tenderness
  ii. Seat-belt mark
    (1) High suspicion for hollow viscous injury

    iii. Penetrating injuries—stab wounds

      (1) Need to rule out peritoneal penetration

        (A) FAST

        (B) Laparoscopy to rule out peritoneal penetration

        (C) Diagnostic peritoneal lavage (commonly replaced by FAST)

    iv. Penetrating injuries—gunshot wounds

      (1) X-rays of abdomen, pelvis, chest to assess for bullets

      (2) Careful examination for wounds

      (3) To the Operating Room for transperitoneal trajectory, peritonitis, hemodynamic instability, hematuria, blood per rectum

      (4) CT scan if stable and suspect extraperitoneal trajectory

  h. Pelvis

    i. Carefully examine perineum, rectum, vagina for lacerations

    ii. Early reduction of dislocated hip

    iii. Early stabilization of pelvis

  i. Back

    i. Examine with patient log-rolled, maintaining spine precautions

  j. Extremities

    i. Gross deformities, wounds, hematomas, tenderness, passive and active range of motion of joints

C. Blood work if not already sent

D. Tetanus, antibiotics if indicated

E. Further tests

  1. CT of head

  2. CT or plain films of C-spine

  3. CT of chest for mechanism of aortic injury

  4. CT of abdomen/pelvis

  5. CT reconstruction of thoracolumbar (T/L) spine or plain films of T/L spine for tenderness or mechanism and unable to examine

  6. Extremity films

F. Tertiary survey

  1. Review all studies, repeat head-to-foot examination, review all laboratory test results for any missed injuries

MENTOR TIPS DIGEST

- The quickest way of ensuring a patent, working airway, as well as a conscious, mentally alert patient, is by getting an appropriate verbal response after asking a patient how he or she is doing.

- In trauma, all patients are considered to have a cervical spinal cord injury and are treated accordingly until it has been proved that no such injury exists. Maintain neck immobilization throughout initial management.

- If the chin lift and jaw thrust fail to establish a patent airway or if the patient is unresponsive, advanced airway intervention with oral endotracheal or nasotracheal intubation is required.

- Three life-threatening ventilatory conditions that must be recognized and treated in the primary survey are tension pneumothorax, open pneumothorax, and flail chest with pulmonary contusion.

- During the primary survey, circulation is assessed by checking three parameters: mental status, skin color, and hemodynamic status (heart rate and blood pressure).

- Hemodynamic instability, defined as heart rate (HR) greater than 100 or systolic blood pressure less than 90, is considered due to blood loss until proved otherwise.

- The classic triad (Beck triad) of hypotension, distended neck veins, and muffled heart sounds is present in fewer than half of patients who are found to have pericardial tamponade.

- The resuscitation phase consists of providing supplemental oxygen, beginning fluid resuscitation with 2 L lactated Ringer solution via two large-bore peripheral IV lines, ECG monitoring, nasogastric tube and Foley insertion, and laboratory evaluation.

- Three x-rays are mandatory in all trauma patients: lateral cervical spine, chest, and pelvis.

- Diagnosis and initial management of pericardial tamponade consist of subxiphoid pericardiocentesis or pericardial window.

Resources

Advanced trauma life support for doctors: Student course manual, 7th ed. American College of Surgeons, 2004.

CDC Injury factbook 2006. Available at http://www.cdc.gov/ncipc/ fact_book/factbook.htm

Hatamabady HR. Mortality in adult patients with blunt injuries in Iran: A comparison of the trauma and injury severity score. Annals of Emergency Medicine 51, 2008.

Jacobs L, Gross R, Luk, S. Advanced trauma operative management. Cinemed Publishers, 2004.

Chapter Self-Test Questions

Circle the correct answer. After you have responded to the questions, check your answers in Appendix A.

1. A patient is tachycardic and tachypneic, with a drop in systolic pressure, altered mental status, and decreased urine output. What is the grade of shock?

   a. Grade I shock, up to 15% blood volume loss

   b. Grade II shock, 15%–30% blood volume loss

   c. Grade III shock, 30%–40% blood volume loss

2. Common causes of injury-related morbidity and mortality rates among patients over age 15 years include all of the following *except:*

   a. Homicide

   b. Suicide

   c. Falls

   d. Motor vehicle crashes

3. Name three x-rays that are mandatory in all trauma patients:

_____

_____

_____

 See the testbank CD for more self-test questions.

BURNS

Manish Tandon, MD

I. Classification and Extent of Burns

A. Types of burns

1. Thermal

    a. Fire

    b. Hot water

    c. Steam

2. Electric

3. Chemical

    a. Acid

    b. Alkali

4. Inhalation

 When in doubt about inhalation injury, intubate.

    a. Tracheobronchitis and edema due to toxic fumes, carbonaceous fumes

    b. Singed nasal/facial hair

    c. Carbonaceous sputum

    d. Hoarse voice

    e. History of a closed-space fire

    f. Direct laryngoscopy, endotracheal intubation

    g. Assume carbon monoxide (CO) toxicity

        i. Check carboxyhemoglobin levels

        ii. Partial pressure of carbon monoxide (pCO) of 1 mm Hg equivalent to carboxyhemoglobin $>40\%$

        iii. Administer 100% Fio_2

        iv. Consider hyperbaric oxygen if altered mental status and no other major injury

B. Levels of burn
   1. Superficial (first degree)
      a. Epidermis only; erythema, pain, no blistering
      b. Red, tender, dry; e.g., sunburn
      c. Heal with topical medications
   2. Partial-thickness (second degree)
      a. Epidermis and dermis
      b. Blisters, weepy, tender
      c. Shallow partial-thickness heal with topical
      d. Deep partial-thickness require débridement
      e. Risk for converting from shallow to deep or to full-thickness
   3. Full-thickness (third degree)
      a. Epidermis and dermis; to muscle, fat, fascia or periosteum; blood vessels, nerve endings destroyed
      b. White/gray/black, dry
      c. Non-tender
      d. Requires débridement
C. Calculating percentage of total body surface area (TBSA) burned
   1. Rule of nines (Table 8.1; Fig. 8.1)

 The rule of nines does not apply to infants and young children.

   2. Using the patient's palm
      a. Full palm, with digits, represents 1% BSA
   3. Does not include superficial burns

TABLE 8.1		
Rule of Nines		
Anatomic Region	**Percentage of TBSA**	
Each arm	9%	(1 nine)
Each leg	18%	(2 nines)
Torso: front	18%	(2 nines)
Torso: back	18%	(2 nines)
Head	9%	(1 nine)

Rule of nines is for adults, not children. The younger the child, the higher percentage of TBSA is the head and lower elsewhere.

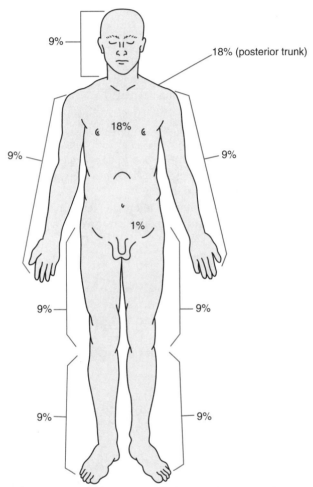

FIGURE 8.1 The rule of nines allows rapid estimation of TBSA covered by burns. Note that with each leg being 18%, upper leg and lower leg can be estimated at 9% each.

II. Initial Assessment and Resuscitation

 Delay in appropriate treatment is the most common cause of complications in severe burn injuries.

A. Many burn injuries present with associated other injuries
B. Airway/breathing

 In burn patients, always start with the ABCs of emergency management.

1. Inhalation injuries
2. Intubation for airway protection, assessment of upper airways
3. Neurologic and disability examinations before intubation when intubation not emergent
4. Fluid resuscitation often exacerbates edema due to airway thermal injury

C. Circulation
1. Fluids
   a. Parkland formula = amount of intravenous (IV) fluid in first 24 hours = weight in kg × 4 mL × percentage BSA burned
      i. Half over first 8 hours
      ii. Half over remaining 16 hours

 Antibiotics are not indicated in the initial burn setting.

   b. Urine output
      i. Maintain urine output (UO) >30 mL/hr
      ii. >100 mL/hr if myoglobinuria present
         (1) Treatment for myoglobinuria: mannitol, hydration, alkalinization of urine with bicarbonate
   c. Over-resuscitation
      i. Compartment syndrome: abdominal, extremity swelling within a closed anatomic compartment (increased pressure in closed compartment causes vascular compromise)
2. Escharotomies
   a. Full-thickness, circumferential burns cause constriction; can prevent perfusion, thoracic expansion, and so on
   b. Treatment by longitudinally incising through thickness of eschar

III. Minimizing Further Damage
A. Tetanus, gastric acid suppression
B. Cooling
  1. Decreases further ischemia of wounds
  2. Caution for hypothermia
C. Management of pain

IV. Topical Antibacterials
A. Silver sulfadiazine (Silvadene)
  1. Initial topical medication for burns
  2. Broad spectrum; not painful
B. Bacitracin
  1. For face, near mucous membranes
  2. Not broad spectrum
C. Mafenide (Sulfamylon)
  1. Penetrates eschars
  2. Painful
  3. Causes acid-base abnormalities

V. Wound Management
A. Early excision and skin grafting
  1. Full-thickness and deep partial-thickness
  2. Tangential excision
  3. Grafting
    a. Autograft
      i. Limited by donor sites
    b. Allograft
      i. Temporary coverage
      ii. Promotes vascularization
    c. Dermis substitute (e.g., Integra) with ultrathin autograft
      i. Monitor for infection
      ii. Structure closer to uninjured skin
    d. Full-thickness autograft
      i. On face and joints
      ii. Donor site longer to heal

VI. Complications

The most common causes of death in burn victims are smoke inhalation injury and infectious complications.

A. Infections (early)
B. Contractures (late)

MENTOR TIPS DIGEST

- When in doubt about inhalation injury, intubate.
- The rule of nines does not apply to infants and young children.
- Delay in appropriate treatment is the most common cause of complications in severe burn injuries.
- In burn patients, always start with the ABCs of emergency management.
- Antibiotics are not indicated in the initial burn setting.
- The most common causes of death in burn victims are smoke inhalation injury and infectious complications.

Resources

Gomez R, Cancio L. Management of burn wounds in the emergency department. Emergency Medicine Clinics of North America 25, 2007.
http://www.nlm.nih.gov/medlineplus/burns.html
Inhalation injury. Available at http://www.emedicine.com/ped/topic1189.htm

Chapter Self-Test Questions

Circle the correct answer. After you have responded to the questions, check your answers in Appendix A.

1. According to the rule of nines, what percentage of total body surface area is represented by each leg?

a. 9%

b. 18%

c. 27%

d. Rule of nines does not apply to legs

2. Which of the following is *not* true of silver sulfadiazine?

   a. Broad-spectrum antibacterial

   b. Initial topical medication for burns

   c. Narrow-spectrum antibacterial

   d. Generally not painful

3. What is a general guideline for how much urine output (UO) you want to maintain with burn patients?

   a. UO <30 mL/hr

   b. UO >20 mL/hr

   c. UO ≤50 mL/hr

   d. UO >30 mL/hr

 See the testbank CD for more self-test questions.

GASTROINTESTINAL HEMORRHAGE

Steven D. Tennenberg, MD

I. Overview

A. Definitions

1. Gastrointestinal (GI)
2. Upper gastrointestinal (UGI): from the esophagus to the ligament of Treitz (junction of fourth portion of duodenum and jejunum)
3. Lower gastrointestinal (LGI): from the ligament of Treitz to the anus

B. Classifications

1. Clinical presentation
   a. Hematemesis
      i. Vomiting bright red blood or bloody material resembling coffee grounds
      ii. UGI source
   b. Hematochezia
      i. Passage of frank blood (bright red blood per rectum [BRBPR]) or bloody or maroon stools
      ii. Usually represents LGI source
   c. Melena
      i. Passage of black tarry stools
      ii. Usually represents UGI source
   d. Occult bleeding
      i. Bleeding detected only by stool guaiac (guaiac-positive) or hemoccult (heme-positive) testing
      ii. Can be UGI or LGI source
2. Acute versus chronic
3. Anatomic source (UGI or LGI)

4. Effect of bleeding on hemodynamic status (vital signs)
    a. Hemodynamically stable
        i. No change in vital signs; no orthostatic changes
        ii. Usually does not require aggressive intravenous (IV) fluid resuscitation
        iii. May or may not require blood transfusions, depending of level of anemia
    b. Hemodynamically unstable
        i. Change in vital signs (heart rate [HR] >100, systolic blood pressure [SBP] <90) or orthostatic changes
        ii. Requires aggressive IV fluid resuscitation
        iii. Usually requires blood transfusions to maintain hemoglobin (Hgb) ≥10 g/dL.
C. Overall algorithm of care
    1. Resuscitation
        a. Two large-bore IVs
        b. Isotonic crystalloid fluid (lactated Ringer or normal saline)
        c. Type and cross for blood transfusions in case needed
        d. Foley catheter to monitor urine output
        e. Serial hemoglobin determinations to assess extent of bleeding and need for transfusions
    2. Evaluation
        a. Nasogastric (NG) tube
            i. Mandatory in serious acute bleeding to rapidly help differentiate UGI from LGI bleeding
            ii. Presence of blood or "coffee ground material" confirms UGI source
            iii. Presence of clear bile very strongly rules out UGI source
            iv. Presence of clear gastric fluid and without bile or blood on lavage with saline strongly rules out UGI source
            v. Allows clearance of blood and gauge of rapidity of bleed in UGI bleeding
        b. Endoscopic: mainstay of definitive diagnosis
            i. Esophagogastroduodenoscopy(EGD): evaluates esophagus, stomach, duodenum; helpful even during active bleeding
            ii. Colonoscopy: evaluates colon; often unhelpful during active bleeding

c. Radiologic
  i. Tagged red blood cell (RBC) study: nuclear medicine study
  ii. Angiography
3. Treatment

 More than 80% of cases stop bleeding spontaneously.

a. Observation
  i. Most (about 80%) acute GI bleeding stops spontaneously.
  ii. Treat underlying cause as indicated.
b. Medical
  i. Antiulcer medication
c. Endoscopic, interventional

 In cases of UGI bleeding, endoscopic therapy is successful more than 80% of the time.

  i. EGD: cauterization, injection
  ii. Colonoscopy: polypectomy, cauterization, injection
d. Radiologic, interventional
  i. Embolization
e. Surgical
  i. For malignant lesions
  ii. For nonmalignant pathology that does not stop bleeding
  iii. Four to six units of blood or more required in fewer than 24 hours
  iv. Rebleeding while hospitalized or readmission for bleeding
D. History
  1. UGI bleeding
    a. Previous history of bleeding and cause
    b. Upper abdominal pain, dyspepsia
    c. Alcohol, nonsteroidal anti-inflammatory drug (NSAID) use
    d. Reflux symptoms
    e. Weight loss, early satiety
    f. Blood dyscrasias, coagulopathies

2. LGI bleeding
   a. Previous history of bleeding and cause
   b. History of diverticulosis
   c. Abdominal pain
   d. Weight loss, change in bowel habits
   e. Diarrhea
   f. History of prostate cancer and radiation therapy (radiation proctitis)
E. Physical examination
   1. UGI bleeding
      a. Abdominal tenderness
      b. Signs of cirrhosis
      c. Abdominal mass
   2. LGI bleeding
      a. Abdominal tenderness
      b. Abdominal mass
      c. Evidence of weight loss

II. Causes of UGI Bleeding (Box 9.1)

 Esophageal, gastric, and colon cancers generally do not cause massive GI bleeding.

BOX 9.1

Ten Most Common and Important Causes of UGI Bleeding

1. Duodenal ulcer/peptic ulcer disease*
2. Gastritis
3. Esophagitis
4. Esophageal varices*
5. Gastric cancer
6. Gastric ulcer
7. Mallory-Weiss tear
8. Esophageal cancer
9. Dieulafoy lesion
10. Aortoenteric fistula

*Most common causes of massive UGI bleeding

A. Duodenal ulcer/peptic ulcer disease
  1. Bleeding usually controlled endoscopically
  2. Medical therapy
    a. H$_2$ blockers
    b. Proton pump inhibitors
    c. Anti–*Helicobacter pylori* therapy
  3. Interventional radiology
    a. Embolization of gastroduodenal artery
    b. For high-risk patients when surgery poor option
  4. Surgical management of bleeding
    a. Oversewing bleeding vessel in ulcer (most patients)
    b. Antiulcer operation in small subset of patients
B. Gastritis
  1. Often associated with alcohol or NSAID use
  2. Usually diffuse in nature so endoscopic management less helpful
  3. Medical therapy with NG lavage and anti-acid therapy usually suffices
C. Esophagitis
  1. Associated with reflux
  2. Bleeding usually responds to anti-acid therapy (proton pump inhibitor preferred)
D. Esophageal varices
  1. Dilated thin veins in distal esophagus due to portal hypertension in cirrhosis
  2. Endoscopic management with banding or injection sclerotherapy optimal
  3. Backup therapy (if endoscopic therapy fails) is use of esophageal balloon tamponade tube (Sengstaken-Blakemore or Minnesota tube), which compresses varices (Fig. 9.1)
  4. Portal venous decompression
    a. Transvenous intrahepatic portosystemic shunt (TIPS)
    b. Operative portosystemic shunt (portocaval or splenorenal shunt) (rare)
E. Gastric cancer
  1. Usually not associated with major bleeding
  2. Definitive management involves gastric resection
  3. If surgery not option, endoscopic lasering or radiation therapy can palliate

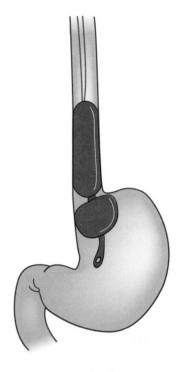

FIGURE 9.1 Correct placement of Sengstaken-Blakemore tube. Note position of gastric and esophageal balloons.

   F. Gastric ulcer
    1. May be peptic in origin
    2. Often associated with NSAID or aspirin use
    3. Bleeding usually controlled endoscopically, allowing medical therapy to heal ulcer
    4. Must rule out malignancy
   G. Mallory-Weiss tear
    1. Mucosal tears in stomach just beyond gastroesophageal junction
    2. Often precipitated by vomiting and retching
    3. Usually stops spontaneously; occasionally requires endoscopic therapy
   H. Esophageal cancer
    1. Often associated with weight loss and dysphagia
    2. Endoscopic lasering can provide some control, radiation therapy for palliation
    3. Management requires surgical resection in appropriate candidates

I. Dieulafoy lesion
      1. Pulsatile arterial vessel in stomach that penetrates through a small mucosal tear
      2. Characterized endoscopically by normal surrounding mucosa
      3. Usually requires endoscopic management
   J. Aortoenteric fistula
      1. Caused by erosion of aortic suture line into duodenum
      2. History of prior aortic surgery with graft
      3. Endoscopy and computed tomography (CT) scanning helpful in diagnosis

III. Causes of LGI Bleeding (Box 9.2)
   A. Diverticulosis
      1. General
         a. Colonic diverticula erode into adjacent bowel wall vessels
         b. Most common cause of significant LGI bleeding
         c. Right-sided diverticula tend to bleed more than left-sided diverticula
         d. Painless
         e. Patient older than 50–60 years
         f. 25% of patients rebleed
         g. History of known diverticula helpful but does not preclude other causes

---

BOX 9.2

Ten Most Common and Important Causes of LGI Bleeding

1. Diverticulosis*
2. Angiodysplasia (arteriovenous malformations)*
3. Colon cancer
4. Inflammatory bowel disease
5. Internal hemorrhoids
6. Radiation proctitis
7. Colon polyps
8. Ischemic colitis
9. Infectious colitis
10. UGI bleeding

*Most common causes of massive LGI bleeding

2. Diagnostic work-up

 Frequently it is difficult to localize the site of a LGI bleed precisely.

  a. Colonoscopy is mainstay
    i. Most commonly diverticulae are seen with luminal blood; no other causes seen
    ii. Occasionally bleeding diverticulum identified
  b. Tagged RBC scan or angiography helpful in localizing side (i.e., right or left colon) of bleeding, which can guide surgery
3. Treatment
  a. Bleeding usually stops spontaneously; no intervention required
  b. Surgery if bleeding does not stop or patient not stabilized
    i. Segmental resection if site/side identified
    ii. Subtotal colectomy if site/side not identified
  c. Surgery for those with recurrent episodes requiring blood transfusions
B. Angiodysplasia (arteriovenous malformations)
  1. Most common in right colon
  2. Isolated bleeding spot can be managed endoscopically
  3. Massive bleeding or chronic intermittent bleeding requires colon resection
C. Colon cancer
  1. Rarely causes massive bleeding
  2. Elective colon resection required after full bowel preparation
D. Inflammatory bowel disease: ulcerative colitis, Crohn disease
  1. Bleeding more common in ulcerative colitis
  2. Bleeding rarely severe enough to require acute surgical intervention
  3. Bleeding usually controlled by medical therapy
E. Internal hemorrhoids
  1. Rarely cause severe bleeding
  2. Typical history of blood on wiping after moving bowels or dripping into toilet bowl
  3. Rule out other causes of colonic bleeding with colonoscopy
F. Radiation proctitis
  1. History of prior prostate radiation
  2. Usually responds to medicated enema therapy

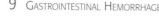

3. More serious and chronic cases may require topical formalin or endoscopic lasering

G. Colon polyps
  1. Large polyps can bleed
  2. Require colonoscopic snare cautery polypectomy

H. Ischemic colitis
  1. Chronic ischemia associated with decreased mesenteric blood flow
  2. Sometimes requires surgical resection of portion of colon

I. Infectious colitis: *Clostridium difficile,* Shigella
  1. History of antibiotic use for *C. difficile* colitis
  2. Shigella associated with foreign travel
  3. Treatment with antibiotics

J. UGI bleeding
  1. Up to 10% of major LGI bleeding from UGI source

IV. Occult GI Bleeding

A. Common causes
  1. Colon cancer
  2. Gastric cancer
  3. Esophageal cancer

B. Clinical presentation
  1. Weight loss
  2. Microcytic, iron-deficiency anemia

V. Small-Bowel Bleeding

A. Accounts for 2%–3% of LGI bleeding

B. Common causes
  1. Meckel diverticulum
  2. Small-bowel tumors
    a. Adenocarcinoma, metastatic or primary
    b. Lymphoma
    c. Capsule or pill endoscopy new diagnostic modality

 MENTOR TIPS DIGEST

- More than 80% of cases stop bleeding spontaneously.
- In cases of UGI bleeding, endoscopic therapy is successful more than 80% of the time.

- Esophageal, gastric, and colon cancers generally do not cause massive GI bleeding.
- Frequently it is difficult to localize the site of a LGI bleed precisely.

Resources

Bounds BC. Lower gastrointestinal bleeding. Gastrointestinal Endoscopy 17:273–288, 2007.

Cappell MS. Initial management of acute upper gastrointestinal bleeding: from initial evaluation up to gastrointestinal endoscopy. Medical Clinics of North America 92:491–509, 2008.

Longacre AV. A commonsense approach to esophageal varices. Clinical Liver Diseases 10:613–625, 2006.

Chapter Self-Test Questions

Circle the correct answer. After you have responded to the questions, check your answers in Appendix A.

1. The most common cause of significant LGI bleeding is:

_____

2. Most common treatment for LGI bleeding is:

_____

3. Bleeding consequent to cancers of the esophagus, stomach, and colon is more often _____ than _____.

4. Typical type of surgery for colon polyps is:

_____

See the testbank CD for more self-test questions.

three

CORE TOPICS

BREAST

Lori L. Wilson, MD, and Mun Jye Poi, MD

I. Benign Breast Disease

A. Pathophysiology

1. The breast is a modified apocrine gland under endocrine control that undergoes continuous change during a woman's lifetime.

2. Constant remodeling of the breast parenchyma is controlled by hormone receptors, genetic aberrations that regulate proliferation and differentiation, and local cellular interactions.

3. Hormonal interactions include paracrine, autocrine, and systemic.

4. Benign epithelial changes of the female breast tissue include nonproliferative lesions, proliferative lesions without atypia, and proliferative lesions with atypical hyperplasia.

5. Most benign parenchymal changes can appear as cystic (fibrocystic change) or nodular lesions (fibroadenoma),

inflammatory changes (acute mastitis or fat necrosis), nipple discharge, or breast pain.

6. Fibroadenomas are composed of stromal and epithelial cells.

   a. Molecular studies demonstrate that fibroadenomas are consistent with hyperplasia and usually grow to less than 3 cm in diameter, remaining constant in size.

7. Following menopause, the decreased influence of hormonal stimulus leads to loss of breast parenchyma, replaced by adipose tissue and often the resolution of benign breast lesions.

8. Nipple discharges are typically physiologic, characteristically bilateral, and clear and nonspontaneous.

B. Epidemiology

1. Benign breast disease includes a heterogeneous group of lesions with incidence increasing during a woman's reproductive life.

2. Breast masses are much more likely to be benign than cancerous.

 Breast masses are much more likely to be benign than cancerous.

3. Most benign lesions are not associated with an increased risk of subsequent breast cancer.

4. Most benign lesions of the breast are inflammatory, stromal, or fibrocystic lesions.

5. Benign proliferative lesions with atypia have a greater risk of breast cancer; these include atypical ductal or lobular hyperplasia.

   a. Less than 20% of patients with a histologic diagnosis of atypical hyperplasia develop invasive cancer during their lifetime.

6. Fibroadenoma is the most frequent benign breast lesion; the peak incidence is between 15 and 35 years of age.

   a. Fibroadenoma is hormone-dependent and most often unilateral.

7. Fibrocystic change, the most common benign symptomatic breast disorder, is most often noted in women younger than 40–50 years old.

   a. It may be bilateral and multifocal.

    b. Up to 50% of women have clinically observed fibrocystic breast changes during their reproductive life.

  8. Inflammatory changes associated with acute mastitis occur more often during the first 3 months following delivery; they result from breastfeeding.

  9. Benign intraductal papilloma, although uncommon, is the most common cause of unilateral, single-duct, bloody, spontaneous nipple discharge.

C. Signs and symptoms

  1. Fibroadenomas are round, smooth, freely mobile, discrete, and spherical.

    a. Typically 1–3 cm in size; may fluctuate in size with menses or oral contraceptive use

    b. Usually solitary and painless

    c. Most often found on breast self-examination

  2. Fibrocystic change is usually multifocal and bilateral.

    a. Tenderness; swelling; focal nodularity

    b. Fluctuates with menstrual cycle; may produce nipple discharge from multiple ducts

  3. Inflammatory changes such as acute mastitis are associated with a painful, cracked nipple.

    a. Breast abscesses usually occur in lactating women.

    b. Abscesses are typically a painful, erythematous, fluctuant mass.

  4. Intraductal papilloma is usually solitary, with discharge emanating from a single duct.

    a. No mass is associated, and discharge is usually bloody.

D. Diagnosis

  1. Medical history and physical examination

  2. Fibroadenoma: mammogram may demonstrate benign, well-circumscribed mass; ultrasound identifies well-circumscribed solid lesion; tissue diagnosis required: core needle biopsy preferred

  3. Fibrocystic change: ultrasound for evaluation of discrete abnormality

    a. Ultrasound-guided fine-needle cyst aspiration

      i. Cysts that fail to resolve or if aspirate bloody: additional work-up for cancer should be performed

4. Intraductal papilloma: ductogram (radiocontrast injection) of involved duct; ductoscopy may identify lesion

5. Lobular carcinoma in situ (LCIS): incidental finding on breast biopsy

E. Management

1. Fibroadenoma: close follow-up with excisional biopsy if lesion changes or patient requests removal

2. Fibrocystic changes: self- and clinical breast examination

a. Consider decreasing xanthines (chocolate, tea, coffee).

b. Consider vitamin E for mild-to-moderate symptoms.

3. Acute mastitis should resolve with appropriate antibiotic therapy; if no resolution: skin biopsy

4. Breast abscess: should be incised, drained

5. Intraductal papilloma should be excised; usually benign and needs no additional treatment

II. Breast Cancer

A. Pathophysiology

1. Ductal carcinoma in situ (DCIS) is proliferation that has not penetrated the basement membrane.

2. LCIS is not cancer; it predicts the future breast cancer in either breast: most commonly invasive ductal carcinoma.

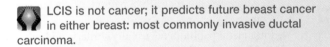

LCIS is not cancer; it predicts future breast cancer in either breast: most commonly invasive ductal carcinoma.

3. Invasive carcinoma of the duct (ductal carcinoma) or lobule (lobular carcinoma) is proliferation of the epithelial cell lining invading the basement membrane.

4. Phyllodes tumors (sarcomas) are cancerous proliferation of stromal origin.

5. LCIS is nonpalpable.

B. Epidemiology

1. During 2007, nearly 181,000 new cases of invasive breast cancer and more than 40,000 breast cancer deaths were estimated in the United States.

Death rates have decreased since 1990, most likely due to improved detection and treatments.

2. One in eight women develop cancer during their lifetime.
3. An increase in noninvasive breast cancer (DCIS) is expected due to screening mammography.
4. Most women diagnosed with breast cancer do not have a known risk factor.
5. Death rates have decreased most likely due to improved detection and treatments.
6. Invasive ductal carcinoma comprises nearly 90% of invasive breast cancers.

 Atypical ductal and lobular hyperplasias are associated with an increased risk of subsequent breast cancer.

7. Tubular, mucinous, papillary, and medullary carcinoma constitute most of the other histologic types.
8. Paget disease, a cutaneous, scaly rash of the nipple, is associated with approximately 3% of breast cancers.
9. Of diagnosed breast cancers, 1% occurs in men.
C. Signs and symptoms
   1. Early-stage breast cancer usually does not produce symptoms when it is small and most treatable.
   2. DCIS is most commonly identified on screening mammography.
      a. Usually nonpalpable
   3. Microcalcifications are clustered with numerous pleomorphic or linear forms (Figs. 10.1 and 10.2).
   4. Invasive ductal carcinoma may be a breast lump found on physical examination (self- or clinical).
   5. Mammographic abnormalities include architectural distortion, asymmetric calcifications, and stellate lesions.
   6. Invasive lobular carcinoma, the most common finding, is a breast mass.
      a. Mammographic abnormality usually noted
   7. Inflammatory breast carcinoma typically presents with an enlarged, indurated, erythematous breast.
      a. Characterized by warmth, edema, skin changes (peau d'orange)
      b. Palpable mass may be associated but not always
      c. Younger women with fairly quick onset
      d. Fails 2-week trial of antibiotics

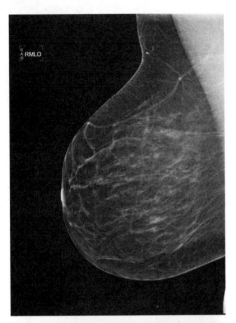

FIGURE 10.1 Normal breast: no calcifications. *(Courtesy of Dr. Mark Kane, Assistant Professor of Radiology, University of Connecticut Health Center, Farmington, Connecticut.)*

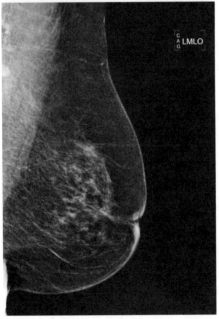

FIGURE 10.2 Breast shows calcifications. *(Courtesy of Dr. Mark Kane, Assistant Professor of Radiology, University of Connecticut Health Center, Farmington, Connecticut.)*

D. Diagnosis

1. DCIS—histologic diagnosis should begin with least invasive biopsy procedure such as stereotactic core-needle biopsy; excisional biopsy if histologic diagnosis discordant

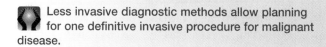

Less invasive diagnostic methods allow planning for one definitive invasive procedure for malignant disease.

2. Invasive ductal or lobular diagnosis—histologic diagnosis by stereotactic or ultrasound-guided core-needle biopsy preferred; excisional biopsy with or without needle localization may also be used

3. Inflammatory breast carcinoma—histologic diagnosis by biopsy for dermal lymphatic involvement; core-needle or excision biopsy of associated mass

4. Cutaneous nipple abnormalities—skin biopsy should be performed; histologic findings of Paget cells should elicit additional evaluation

E. Management

1. Ductal carcinoma in situ (noninvasive breast cancer) requires only partial mastectomy with negative margins; nodal evaluation not necessary

    a. Postoperative radiation is necessary for DCIS greater than 1 cm

2. Invasive breast cancer staging to include tumor size, lymph node status, evidence of distant metastasis

    a. Axillary node status excellent prognostic indicator for invasive breast cancer with positive nodes indicating systemic disease

    b. Sentinel node biopsy performed by radiolabeled colloid and blue dye with subareolar or parenchymal injection for invasive breast cancer; sentinel node is first draining lymph node: located using a gamma probe prior to incision and direct visualization of blue node following incision; sentinel node excised and evaluated pathologically; if positive: axillary lymph node dissection indicated; randomized studies evaluating if axillary lymph node dissection necessary

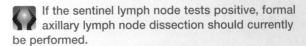

If the sentinel lymph node tests positive, formal axillary lymph node dissection should currently be performed.

c. Breast cancer less than 4 cm: breast-conserving surgery may be performed, including atrial mastectomy (lumpectomy) with 1-cm margins followed by 4500 Gray postoperative radiation; mastectomy may also be performed, surgically resecting all breast tissue; neoadjuvant chemotherapy may be considered for cancers greater than 2 cm

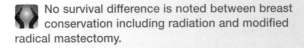

Radiation is for local control, and chemotherapy is used for systemic control.

d. For axillary lymph involvement, formal axillary lymph node dissection of levels I and II performed
e. Mastectomy with formal axillary lymph node dissection is modified radical mastectomy

No survival difference is noted between breast conservation including radiation and modified radical mastectomy.

f. Modified radical mastectomy may be followed by immediate breast reconstruction
g. Axillary radiation is alternative to formal axillary dissection
h. Hormonal therapy using antiestrogen drugs such as tamoxifen reduces recurrence, improves survival in DCIS and estrogen and progesterone receptor-positive tumors
i. Chemotherapy indicated for positive lymph nodes, aggressive histologic or molecular markers with tumors greater than 1 cm
j. Multidrug chemotherapies include cyclophosphamide, Adriamycin, or methotrexate, 5-fluorouracil.
3. Inflammatory breast carcinoma and large locally invasive breast cancers usually first treated with chemotherapy
   a. Radiation for local control; chemotherapy for systemic control

F. Survival
  1. Table 10.1 lists average survival rates.

 Combined 5-year survival rates for invasive breast cancer is 88%.

G. Prevention
  1. Although there are no sure ways to prevent breast cancer, choose lifestyle habits such as maintaining healthy diet, engaging regular exercise, avoiding obesity, eliminating tobacco use, limiting alcohol consumption, and considering the risk of hormone replacement therapy.
  2. Breast cancer screening can detect breast lesions needing further evaluation and identify smaller, more localized breast cancers.
  3. Two-thirds of breast cancers are diagnosed at an early stage by mammographic screening.
  4. Approximately 70% of eligible women (40 years and older) had a mammogram between 1998 and 2000.
  5. The American Cancer Society recommends screening (asymptomatic) mammograms beginning at age 40 years.
  6. Clinical breast examination by a health-care provider should occur at least every 3 years from age 20 years and yearly after age 40.
  7. Women at increased risk should be considered for earlier screening before age 40 years.
  8. Digital mammography is significantly better in screening women younger than 50 years or women of any age with dense breasts.

TABLE 10.1	
Breast Cancer Survival Rates	
Stage	Rate
Stage I	98%
Stage II	89%
Stage III	80%
Stage IV	26%

H. History and physical examination

1. Complete medical history is required of any patient with symptomatic breast disease.

2. Medical history allows assessment of patient's risk of breast cancer.

3. Risk factor assessment includes age, inherited genetic mutations (*BRCA-1* or *BRCA-2*), personal or family history of breast cancer, personal or family history of ovarian cancer, biopsy-proven atypical hyperplasia, high breast density, reproductive factors (early menarche, late menopause, nulliparity), and long-term use of hormone replacement therapy.

4. Physical examination includes inspection and palpation in both the sitting and supine position.

   a. Inspection includes arms at the side, above the head, and firmly pressing at the waist; assessing skin dimpling or superficial cutaneous changes, breast symmetry or edema, and nipple retraction or inversion.

   b. Cervical, supraclavicular, and axillary lymph nodes are palpated.

5. Examination of the breast includes palpation to identify parenchymal changes.

   a. Changes of texture, size, contour, tenderness, fixation, and mobility along with location are noted.

6. Findings suggestive of cancer include a hard or painless breast mass, unilateral breast enlargement, skin changes (dimpling or redness), and enlarged lymph nodes that are firm, fixed, or painless.

7. Nipple discharge is noted along with its character and color; bloody is most likely associated with intraductal papilloma more rarely than cancer, green or brown fluid is related to fibrocystic change, milky discharge.

I. Differential diagnosis

1. Radiographic evaluation

   a. Standard screening mammography involves a two-view (craniocaudal, mediolateral) x-ray of asymptomatic breasts.

   b. Diagnostic mammography includes an initial two-view x-ray and additional views (i.e., oblique, magnified, or compression) to further evaluate additional abnormalities.

   i. False-negative rate 5%–10%

    c. Most common abnormal mammographic findings are dominant masses and microcalcification.

        i. Microcalcifications characterized by number and morphology

    d. Ultrasonography is a noninvasive tool for mammography-detected abnormalities or palpable masses.

        i. Not utilized as a screening tool but useful in delineating solid versus cystic breast masses

        ii. Also useful for younger and pregnant women

J. Biopsy techniques

  1. Diagnosis is made by histologic evaluation.

    a. Samples are taken by core-needle, incisional, or excisional biopsy.

  2. Preferred method for diagnosis of a palpable solid mass is core-needle biopsy.

  3. Nonpalpable breast lesions diagnosis may utilize guidance (stereotactic or ultrasound) for core-needle biopsy on lesions that are only radiographically identifiable.

    a. If core-needle biopsy cannot establish the diagnosis, needle localization biopsy is used.

  4. Less invasive diagnostic methods allow planning for one definitive invasive procedure for malignant disease.

  5. Pathologic evaluation includes histologic evaluation by hematoxylin and eosin (H&E) stain, with evidence of malignancy estrogen and progesterone receptor and *her-2-neu* status, is assessed.

Resources

Abeloff M. Abeloff's clinical oncology, 4th ed. Churchill Livingstone, 2008.

Newman LA, Mamounas EP. Review of breast cancer clinical trials conducted by the national surgical adjuvant breast project. Surgical Clinics of North America 87, 2007.

MENTOR TIPS DIGEST

- Breast masses are much more likely to be benign than cancer.
- LCIS is not cancer; it predicts future breast cancer in either breast: most commonly invasive ductal carcinoma.
- Death rates have decreased since 1990, most likely due to improved detection and treatments.
- Atypical ductal and lobular hyperplasias are associated with an increased risk of subsequent breast cancer.
- Less invasive diagnostic methods allow planning for one definitive invasive procedure for malignant disease.
- If the sentinel lymph node tests positive, formal axillary lymph node dissection should currently be performed.
- Radiation is for local control, and chemotherapy is used for systemic control.
- No survival difference is noted between breast conservation including radiation and modified radical mastectomy.
- Combined 5-year survival rates for invasive breast cancer is 88%.

Chapter Self-Test Questions

Circle the correct answer. After you have responded to the questions, check your answers in Appendix A.

1. _____ is the most frequent benign breast lesion.

2. Which type of biopsy is the preferred method for diagnosis of a palpable solid mass?

_____

3. List five risk factors for breast cancer:

_____

_____

_____

_____

_____

See the testbank CD for more self-test questions.

11

THYROID AND PARATHYROIDS

Robert A. Kozol, MD

I. Anatomy
A. Location and relationships
1. Thyroid is draped over trachea
2. From superficial to deep (anterior to posterior) thyroid, trachea, cervical esophagus, vertebral column

B. Blood supply
1. Superior thyroid arteries (left and right): from external carotid arteries
2. Inferior thyroid arteries (left and right): from thyrocervical trunk

C. Nerves
1. Recurrent laryngeal nerves (left and right) from vagus nerves; innervate all laryngeal muscles except cricothyroid muscle

> The recurrent laryngeal nerves, the branches of the vagus that innervate the muscles of the larynx, run in the tracheoesophageal groove on each side of the neck. Injury to a recurrent nerve causes a permanent voice change, usually hoarseness.

2. External branch of superior laryngeal nerve innervates cricothyroid muscle

II. Thyroid Cancer
A. Pathophysiology
1. Activation of receptor tyrosine kinases *(RET/PTC):* may be radiation-induced
2. Somatic point mutations (*BRAF* gene)

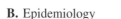

B. Epidemiology
  1. 30,000 new cases per year in United States
  2. Female/male ratio is 2.5/1
  3. Cell types
    a. Papillary carcinoma 75%
    b. Follicular carcinoma 15%
    c. Medullary carcinoma 5%
    d. Anaplastic carcinoma less than 5%
C. Prevention
  1. Avoid radiation to the neck
D. History and physical examination
  1. Signs and symptoms of hypo- or hyperthyroidism
  2. Family history of thyroid tumors
  3. Family history of multiple endocrine neoplasia II (MEN II)
  4. History of cervical radiation
    a. External beam to neck
    b. Nuclear accident
  5. Voice change
  6. Thyroid nodule found on examination (Fig. 11.1)
    a. Have patient swallow: thyroid nodule moves vertically on swallowing; other neck lumps do not

 A thyroid nodule can be differentiated from other central neck masses by the fact that a thyroid nodule moves up and down with swallowing.

  7. Check for lymphadenopathy (neck)
E. Differential diagnosis
  1. Thyroid cancer
  2. Benign thyroid nodule
  3. Multinodular goiter
  4. Non-thyroid neck mass
F. Management
  1. Surgical resection
    a. Cancer 1 cm or smaller requires only lobectomy and isthmusectomy.
    b. Cancer greater than 1-cm diameter requires total or near-total thyroidectomy.

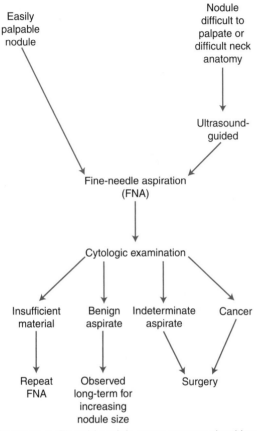

Figure 11.1 Thyroid nodule management algorithm.

i. Total thyroidectomy: attempt to remove 100% of the gland; near-total thyroidectomy: small bits of thyroid parenchyma left to preserve nerves and parathyroids

ii. Postoperative radioactive iodine to obliterate any residual thyroid tissue in neck

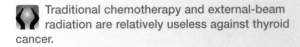

Traditional chemotherapy and external-beam radiation are relatively useless against thyroid cancer.

    iii. Goal: negative total body thyroid scan, serum thyroglobulin level of 0
    iv. Allows for follow-up with total body thyroid scans, serum thyroglobulin levels as tests for recurrent or metastatic disease
  c. Complications of thyroidectomy
    i. Permanent voice change (recurrent laryngeal nerve [RLN] injury): 3%
    ii. Neck hematoma requiring reoperation: 1%
    iii. Permanent hypoparathyroidism (severe hypocalcemia): 5%–8%
G. Prognosis
  1. Papillary cancer greater than 90% cure rate with surgery
  2. Follicular cancer
    a. Noninvasive variant (common) greater than 90% cure rate with surgery
    b. Invasive variant, deaths due to metastatic disease seen 5–15 years later
  3. Medullary cancer
    a. 50% of patients are node-negative, yielding a greater than 90% cure rate with surgery
    b. 50% of patients are node-positive, leading to deaths seen during follow-up over years
  4. Anaplastic cancer
    a. Invades trachea, esophagus, bone
    b. Uniformly fatal (no effective treatment)
  5. Prognostic factors
    a. Cell type (papillary best, anaplastic worst)
    b. Age (under 45 years: better; over 45 years: poorer)
    c. Size (smaller than 5 cm: better; larger than 5 cm: poorer)
    d. Gender (women do slightly better than men)

III. Hyperparathyroidism

A. Pathophysiology
  1. Elevated parathyroid hormone
    a. Increased calcium mobilized from bone
    b. Increased calcium absorption in gastrointestinal (GI) tract
    c. Increased serum calcium level
  2. Secondary and tertiary hyperparathyroidism
    a. Both in context of chronic renal failure

    b. Almost always four-gland hyperplasia

    c. Tertiary hyperparathyroidism involves four autonomous glands (the parathyroid [PTH] level stays very high regardless of serum calcium level)

B. Epidemiology

  1. 85% solitary adenoma

  2. 15% four-gland hyperplasia

C. Signs and symptoms

  1. Severe cases: "moans, bones, and stones" (psychiatric moans, bone thinning, kidney stones)

  2. Less severe cases:

    a. Joint pain

    b. Weakness

    c. Fatigue

    d. Anxiety

    e. Memory loss

D. History and physical examination

  1. Ask about symptoms listed above

  2. Examine neck

    a. Parathyroid glands (normal or enlarged are not palpable)

    b. Looking for other disorder (e.g., thyroid nodules, nodes, etc.)

E. Differential diagnosis

  1. Most cases incidentally picked up as hypercalcemia on routine blood tests

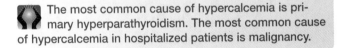 The most common cause of hypercalcemia is primary hyperparathyroidism. The most common cause of hypercalcemia in hospitalized patients is malignancy.

    a. Hypercalcemia of malignancy

      i. PTH level normal, parathyroid hormone-related peptide (PTHrP) elevated

      ii. Usually associated with bone metastases from other cancers

    b. Milk-alkali syndrome (too much calcium intake)

    c. Familial hypocalciuric hypercalcemia

F. Management

  1. Preoperative parathyroid (sestamibi) nuclear scan

  2. Second-line test: cervical ultrasonography

3. If adenoma localized by scan, operative therapy is removal of enlarged gland (focused, minimally invasive approach) with pre- and post-removal rapid PTH assay in the operating room

 With parathyroid exploration, the disorder is determined by examining the size of each gland with the naked eye. Parathyroids larger than 8 mm in their greatest dimension are abnormal

    a. If successful, PTH should drop by more than 50% and in the normal range 10 min after excision

4. If sestamibi negative or suggests multiple-gland disease, formal neck exploration recommended

5. If four-gland hyperplasia found, three and one-half gland resection indicated:

    a. MEN syndromes

      i. Men I

      ii. Pancreatic islet cell tumor

      iii. Pituitary adenoma

      iv. Parathyroid hyperplasia

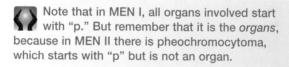 Note that in MEN I, all organs involved start with "p." But remember that it is the *organs*, because in MEN II there is pheochromocytoma, which starts with "p" but is not an organ.

The rapid PTH test works because the half-life of PTH is 2–3 minutes.

TABLE 11.1	
Comparison of MEN IIA and MEN IIB	
MEN IIA	**MEN IIB**
Pheochromocytoma	Pheochromcytoma
Medullary carcinoma thyroid	MCT
Parathyroid hyperplasia	No para hyper; instead, soft-tissue tumors and other findings

MENTOR TIPS DIGEST

- The recurrent laryngeal nerves, the branches of the vagus that innervate the muscles of the larynx, run in the tracheoesophageal groove on each side of the neck. Injury to a recurrent nerve causes a permanent voice change, usually hoarseness.
- A thyroid nodule can be differentiated from other central neck masses by the fact that a thyroid nodule moves up and down with swallowing.
- Traditional chemotherapy and external-beam radiation are relatively useless against thyroid cancer.
- The most common cause of hypercalcemia is primary hyperparathyroidism. The most common cause of hypercalcemia in hospitalized patients is malignancy.
- With parathyroid exploration, the disorder is determined by examining the size of each gland with the naked eye. Parathyroids larger than 8 mm in their greatest dimension are abnormal.
- Note that in MEN I, all organs involved start with "p." But remember that it is the *organs*, because in MEN II there is pheochromocytoma, which starts with "p" but is not an organ.
- The rapid PTH test works because the half-life of PTH is 2–3 minutes.

Resources

Coker LH, Rorie K, Cantley L, et al. Primary hyperparathyroidism, cognition, and health-related quality of life. Annals of Surgery 242:642–650, 2005.

Dackiw AP, Zeiger M. Extent of surgery for differentiated thyroid cancer. Surgical Clinics of North America. 84:817–832, 2004.

Chapter Self-Test Questions

Circle the correct answer. After you have responded to the questions, check your answers in Appendix A.

1. List three complications of thyroidectomy:

_____

_____

_____

2. Which nerves innervate all laryngeal muscles except the cricothyroid muscle?

_____

3. In the surgical resection of thyroid cancer, cancer >1-cm diameter requires total or near-total thyroidectomy; cancer 1 cm or smaller requires only _____

See the testbank CD for more self-test questions.

12

ACUTE ABDOMEN AND APPENDICITIS

Robert A. Kozol, MD

I. Acute Abdomen

A. Types of pain (Table 12.1)

1. Visceral pain
   a. Poorly localized
   b. Occurs centrally in three zones (epigastric, periumbilical, suprapubic)
   c. Zone of presentation depends on organ(s) involved and arterial blood supply
      i. Organs with celiac trunk–derived blood supply: epigastric pain
      ii. Superior mesenteric artery: periumbilical pain
      iii. Inferior mesenteric artery: suprapubic pain
2. Parietal pain
   a. Well localized
   b. Localized by inflamed organ irritating parietal peritoneum

TABLE 12.1	Types of Abdominal Pain	
	Visceral	**Parietal**
Character	Vague	
	May be crampy	Sharp
Location	Toward midline	
	Poorly localized	Anywhere in abdomen
Noxious stimuli	Ischemia or smooth muscle stretch (distention)	Infection or inflammation

    c. Usually identified by quadrant: right upper (RUQ), right lower (RLQ), left upper (LUQ), left lower (LLQ)

    d. Quadrants have common inflammatory diseases

        i. RUQ: acute cholecystitis

        ii. RLQ: acute appendicitis

        iii. LLQ: acute sigmoid diverticulitis

B. Peritonitis

  1. May be localized or diffused

  2. Detected on physical examination

    a. Involuntary guarding

    b. Rebound tenderness

  3. Common cause: perforated viscus

    a. "Free air" seen on plain film or computed tomography (CT) scan

> Free intraperitoneal air is most common with a perforated peptic ulcer and is less common with perforated appendicitis or perforated sigmoid diverticulitis.

  4. Requires fluid resuscitation and emergency surgery

C. Common causes

  1. Visceral pain

    a. Early appendicitis

    b. Small-bowel obstruction

    c. Large-bowel obstruction

    d. Biliary colic

    e. Intestinal ischemia

  2. Parietal pain

    a. Late appendicitis

    b. Acute cholecystitis

    c. Sigmoid diverticulitis (microperforation)

    d. Pelvic inflammatory disease

  3. Peritonitis

    a. Perforated peptic ulcer

    b. Sigmoid diverticulitis (macroperforation)

    c. Intestinal ischemia with intestinal necrosis

    d. Other bowel perforations

D. History
   1. Mnemonic for interviewing patients with pain: PQRST
      a. P: palliative/provocative factor
      b. Q: quality
      c. R: radiation
      d. S: severity
      e. T: temporal sequence

> ⚡ Two situations suggest disease of a surgical nature: abdominal pain that persists beyond 6 hours and abdominal pain that is severe and began so suddenly that the patient noted the exact time.

> ⚡ Severe abdominal pain out of proportion to physical findings suggests mesenteric ischemia (this is an emergency).

E. Physical examination
   1. Inspection
   2. Auscultation (silent abdomen may be peritonitis)
   3. Palpation/percussion
      a. Diffuse tenderness, rebound, guarding is peritonitis, likely requiring operation

II. Acute Appendicitis

A. Pathophysiology
   1. Obstruction of appendiceal lumen
      a. In babies and very young children from lymphoid hyperplasia in wall of appendix
      b. In adults from fecalith
B. Epidemiology
   1. Can occur in any age group but more common in ages 16–30 years
C. Prevention
   1. Nonapplicable
D. Signs and symptoms
   1. Begins as periumbilical pain (visceral pain due to obstruction of hollow viscus)
   2. Pain shifting to RLQ as inflamed appendix irritates parietal peritoneum (parietal pain)

3. On examination significant RLQ tenderness
4. Rovsing sign: when palpation of LLQ results in pain in RLQ
5. Obturator sign: raise patient's right leg with knee flexed; rotate leg internally at hip; increased abdominal pain indicates positive sign
6. Psoas sign: place your hand above patient's right knee; have patient flex right hip against resistance; increased abdominal pain indicates positive sign

E. History and physical examination
   1. Begins with vague periumbilical pain
   2. Nausea and vomiting may follow but rarely precede onset of pain
   3. Anorexia common
   4. Pain shift to RLQ
   5. On examination RLQ tender

F. Differential diagnosis
   1. Gastroenteritis (patients usually develop diarrhea)
   2. Cecal diverticulitis
   3. Typhlitis (cecal inflammation in immunosuppressed patients)
   4. Mesenteric lymphadenitis
   5. Ruptured ovarian cyst (right)
   6. Ovarian torsion (right)
   7. Ruptured ectopic pregnancy (right)
   8. Pelvic inflammatory disease (females only)

> Beware of "crossover" diseases: e.g., myocardial infarction (MI) causing epigastric pain, right lower leg pneumonia presenting with RUQ pain, sigmoid colon flopped into RLQ mimicking appendicitis

G. Management
   1. Workup includes complete blood count (CBC); pregnancy test if applicable; if clinical picture is "classic" (males): appendectomy (open or laparoscopic) otherwise perform CT scan
   2. CT scanning, if result positive, leads to surgery (greater than 90% accuracy); if negative, leads to discharge or observation
   3. Appendectomy by laparoscopic or open technique
   4. If perforated, may need 3–7 days of intravenous antibiotics

5. Neglected appendicitis is a perforation 3–5 days old with abscess or mass
   a. Treated with IR placed drain and intravenous antibiotics
   b. Interval appendectomy 2 months later remains controversial

 MENTOR TIPS DIGEST

- Free intraperitoneal air is most common with a perforated peptic ulcer and is less common with perforated appendicitis or perforated sigmoid diverticulitis.
- Two situations suggest disease of a surgical nature: abdominal pain that persists beyond 6 hours and abdominal pain that is severe and began so suddenly that the patient noted the exact time.
- Severe abdominal pain out of proportion to physical findings suggests mesenteric ischemia (this is an emergency).
- Beware of "crossover" diseases: e.g., myocardial infarction (MI) causing epigastric pain, RLL pneumonia presenting with RUQ pain, sigmoid colon flopped into RLQ mimicking appendicitis.

Resources

Silen W, ed: Cope's early diagnosis of the acute abdomen. Oxford University Press, 2007.

Townsend CM: Sabiston textbook of surgery, 18th ed. WB Saunders, 2007.

Chapter Self-Test Questions

Circle the correct answer. After you have responded to the questions, check your answers in Appendix A.

1. What conditions can mask abdominal pain associated with the acute abdomen?

   a. Steroids

   b. Diabetes

   c. Narcotics

   d. All of the above

2. What test should every woman of childbearing age with an acute abdomen receive?

a. Serum amylase

b. Urinalysis

c. B-HCG

d. AFP

3. Which of the following causes abdominal pain out of proportion to the examination?

a. Mesenteric ischemia

b. Pancreatitis

c. PID

d. Cystitis

4. What percentage of the population will develop appendicitis sometime during their life?

a. 15%

b. 7%

c. 25%

d. 33%

5. What condition causes pain limited to specific dermatomes?

a. Testicular torsion

b. Kidney stone

c. Early zoster before vesicles erupt

d. Pancreatitis

See the testbank CD for more self-test questions.

13
CHAPTER

STOMACH
AND DUODENUM

Robert A. Kozol, MD, and Tamar Lipof, MD

I. Anatomy

  A. Location

    1. Stomach

      a. Upper abdomen

      b. Gastroesophageal junction is intra-abdominal

      c. Adjacent to spleen on patient's left

      d. Adjacent to liver on patient's right

    2. Duodenum

      a. Four portions forming C-loop

      b. Head of pancreas sits inside the C-loop

      c. Posterior surface retroperitoneal

  B. Blood supply

    1. Stomach

      a. Left gastric artery (from celiac trunk)

      b. Right gastric artery (from common hepatic artery)

      c. Left gastroepiploic artery (from splenic artery)

      d. Right gastroepiploic artery (from gastroduodenal artery)

      e. Short gastric arteries (from splenic artery)

    2. Duodenum

      a. Gastroduodenal artery

      b. Shared blood supply with head of pancreas

  C. Vagus nerves

    1. Vagi are left and right in thorax

    2. Become anterior and posterior in abdomen (pneumonic: LARP [left/anterior, right/posterior])

II. Peptic Ulcer Disease
A. Pathophysiology

 The two most common ulcerogenics are *H. pylori* and NSAIDs.

   1. Infectious disease
   a. *Helicobacter pylori* (pathogen)
   i. Lives in gastric antrum
   2. Drug-induced
   a. Nonsteroidal anti-inflammatory drugs (NSAIDs)
   i. Direct mucosal injury
   3. Gastric acid hypersecretion
   a. Non–*H. pylori*, non-NSAID ulcer
   b. Gastrinoma
   i. Islet cell tumor of pancreas or duodenum
   ii. Secretes gastrin, which stimulates gastric acid secretion
   iii. Causes severe ulcer diathesis (Zollinger-Ellison syndrome)
   iv. Multiple ulcers
   v. Ectopic ulcers
   vi. Diarrhea
B. Epidemiology
   1. Incidence of peptic ulcer has been declining for more than 50 years
   2. Incidence of complications of ulcers (hemorrhage and perforation) has remained stable
   3. Peptic ulcer: *H. pylori* association
   a. Duodenal ulcer: 80%–90% *H. pylori*–positive
   b. Gastric ulcer: 70% *H. pylori*–positive
C. Prevention
   1. Good hygiene
   2. Avoid NSAIDs
   3. Avoid smoking
D. Signs and symptoms
   1. Epigastric pain (dyspepsia)
   2. Nausea and vomiting
   3. Upper gastrointestinal (GI) bleeding

E. History and physical examination
  1. History of risk factors
  2. History of epigastric pain, nausea, sometimes emesis
  3. Pain often relieved with food or antacids
  4. No reliable physical findings
F. Differential diagnosis
  1. Gastritis
  2. Cholelithiasis
  3. Pancreatitis
  4. Gastroesophageal reflux (GERD)
  5. Gastric cancer
G. Management
  1. Diagnosis confirmed by esophagogastroduodenoscopy (EGD)
  2. H_2-receptor blockade (ranitidine)
  3. Proton pump inhibitors
  4. If patient is *H. pylori*–positive: eradicate *H. pylori*
  5. Surgery for complicated peptic ulcer (Table 13.1)

 Perforated gastric or duodenal ulcers are surgical emergencies.

  a. For perforation: perform Graham patch (omental flap laid over perforation and sutured in place)
  b. For hemorrhage (usually gastroduodenal artery) posterior ulcer in first position of duodenum: open anterior duodenal

TABLE 13.1			
Comparisons of Antiulcer Operations			
Operation	Recurrence Rate	Complication Rate (Including Dumping)	
Parietal cell vagotomy (highly selective vagotomy)	About 10%	Low	(<10%)
Vagotomy and emptying procedure (pyloroplasty or gastrojejunostomy)	5%–10%	Intermediate	(10%–15%)
Vagotomy and antrectomy	2%–3%	High	(15%–25%)

wall with incision through pylorus; over-sew gastroduodenal artery and close duodenum as a pyloroplasty; consider truncal vagotomy (bilateral)
  c. For gastric outlet obstruction
    i. If inflammatory: conservative management (nasogastric tube + H_2 blockers)
    ii. If fibrotic—surgical therapy

III. Gastric Adenocarcinoma
A. Pathophysiology
  1. Risk factors
    a. Atrophic gastritis
    b. Pernicious anemia
    c. Gastric polyps
    d. *H. pylori* infection
    e. Diet high in nitrates
    f. Asian ethnicity
B. Epidemiology
  1. Declining incidence of gastric cancer for many decades
  2. Approximately 22,000 new cases in United States per year
  3. Proximal gastric cancers more common than distal cancers
C. Prevention
  1. Avoid smoke-preserved and salt-cured foods
  2. Eradication of *H. pylori*
D. Signs and symptoms
  1. No early signs or symptoms
  2. Late symptoms
    a. Early satiety
    b. Weight loss
    c. Epigastric pain
E. History and physical examination
  1. History of *H. pylori* infection, gastric polyps, atrophic gastritis
  2. History of early satiety and weight loss
  3. Late signs on physical examination
    a. Epigastric mass
    b. Left supraclavicular adenopathy (Virchow node)
F. Differential diagnosis
  1. Peptic ulcer disease
  2. Pancreatic cancer

3. Gastric lymphoma
4. Gastrointestinal stromal tumor

G. Management
1. EGD with biopsies

> Because of the chance of malignancy, the rim of all gastric ulcers should be biopsied when they are identified endoscopically (do not biopsy duodenal ulcers).

2. Computed tomography (CT) scanning
3. Endoscopic ultrasound
4. Mainstay of therapy—surgical resection (partial or total gastrectomy) (Figs. 13.1, 13.2, 13.3)
5. If patient has widespread metastases: palliative care

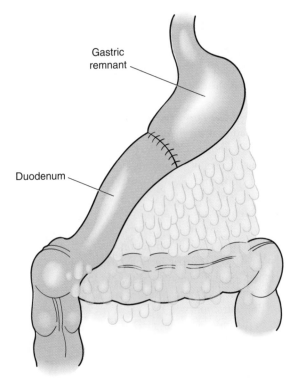

Gastric remnant

Duodenum

FIGURE 13.1 Billroth I reconstruction after partial gastrectomy.

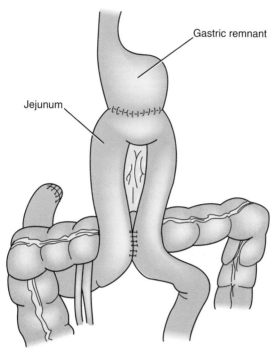

Gastric remnant

Jejunum

FIGURE 13.2 Billroth II gastrojejunostomy after partial gastrectomy. Note that the duodenal stump is oversewn.

6. Combined regional radiation therapy plus 5-fluorouracil and leucovorin given postoperatively may prolong survival

7. Extent of lymph-node dissection with gastrectomy

    a. D0—immediate juxta-gastric nodes only

    b. D1—nodes along hepatic, splenic, gastric arteries

    c. D2—includes celiac nodes

    d. D3—includes para-aortic nodes

H. Outcomes

> The two most important prognostic factors in gastric cancer are depth of gastric wall invasion and lymph node status.

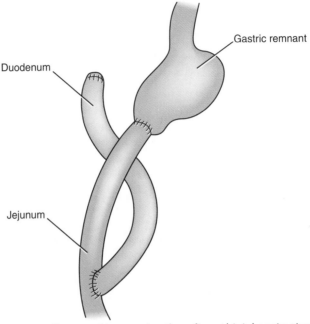

FIGURE 13.3 Roux-en-Y reconstruction after subtotal gastrectomy.

1. Survival by stage after surgery (5 years)
   a. $T_1 N_0$—90%
   b. $T_2 N_0$—50%
   c. $T_3 N_0$—40%
   d. Any $T N_1$—20%
   e. Distant metastases—approaches 0

MENTOR TIPS DIGEST
- The two most common ulcerogenics are *H. pylori* and NSAIDs.
- Perforated gastric or duodenal ulcers are surgical emergencies.
- Because of the chance of malignancy, the rim of all gastric ulcers should be biopsied when they are identified endoscopically (do not biopsy duodenal ulcers).
- The two most important prognostic factors in gastric cancer are depth of gastric wall invasion and lymph node status.

Resources

Khan FA, Shukla AN. Pathogenesis and treatment of gastric carcinoma: An up-date with brief review. Journal of Cancer Research & Therapeutics 2:196–199, 2006.

Lipof T, Shapiro D, Kozol RA. Surgical perspectives in peptic ulcer disease and gastritis. World Journal of Gastroenterology 12:3248–3252, 2006.

Martin RF. Surgical management of ulcer disease. Surgical Clinics of North America 85:907–929, 2005.

Chapter Self-Test Questions

Circle the correct answer. After you have responded to the questions, check your answers in Appendix A.

1. All of the following arteries are branches off the celiac trunk *except:*

   a. Left gastric artery

   b. Splenic artery

   c. Common hepatic artery

   d. Left gastroepiploic artery

2. Which infectious agent is associated with peptic ulcer disease?

   a. *Haemophilus influenzae*

   b. *Helicobacter pylori*

   c. *Staphylococcus aureus*

   d. *Haemophilus ducreyi*

3. All of the following are true about gastrinomas *except:*

   a. They may be found in MEN type I patients.

   b. They may be found in MEN type II patients.

   c. They are associated with significantly elevated gastrin levels.

   d. The diarrhea that results can be halted by aspiration of gastric secretions.

4. The artery most often responsible for upper GI bleeding associated with duodenal ulcers is the:

   a. Gastroduodenal artery

   b. Right gastric artery

   c. Right gastroepiploic artery

   d. Superior mesenteric artery

5. Indications for surgical treatment of a peptic ulcer include all of the following *except:*

   a. Gastric outlet obstruction due to peptic ulcer disease

   b. Peptic ulcer disease refractory to medical treatment

   c. *H. pylori* infection associated with peptic ulcer disease

   d. Perforation due to peptic ulcer disease

   e. Bleeding duodenal ulcer that has failed endoscopic therapy

See the testbank CD for more self-test questions.

14

HEPATOBILIARY SYSTEM

Yuri W. Novitsky, MD, and Mun Jye Poi, MD

I. Liver

  A. Anatomy

    1. Largest solid organ in the body

    2. Located in right upper quadrant (RUQ)

    3. Attachments

      a. Coronary ligaments (anterior and posterior)

        i. Formed by reflections of peritoneum

        ii. Leaves of coronary ligaments combine to form left and right triangular ligaments

      b. Falciform ligament

        i. Formed by anterior layer of coronary ligament

        ii. Extends between liver and anterior abdominal wall

        iii. Contains remnant of embryonic left umbilical vein (round ligament)

      c. Gastrohepatic ligament (lesser omentum)

      d. Hepatoduodenal ligament

        i. Contains hepatic artery, portal vein, and common bile duct

    4. Morphology

      a. Divided into two lobes by imaginary plane from vena cava to gallbladder (GB) bed

        i. Right lobe

          (1) Posterior and anterior segments

        ii. Left lobe

          (1) Medial and lateral segments (separated by falciform ligament)

        iii. Caudate lobe

     5. Blood supply

       a. Hepatic artery (from celiac trunk)

         i. Right and left branches

       b. Portal vein

         i. Confluence of superior mesenteric and splenic veins

         ii. Divides into right and left branches

B. Physiology

     1. Filtration and detoxification function

     2. Glycogen production and storage

     3. Phospholipid and cholesterol synthesis

     4. Conjugation of bilirubin

     5. Protein and clotting factors synthesis

       a. Albumin and ProTime are best markers of liver function

       b. Liver failure manifests by disorders of filtration and/or synthetic functions (Table 14.1)

 The most common cause of liver failure requiring transplantation in the United States is hepatitis C.

C. Pathophysiology

     1. Hepatic abscess

       a. Classification

         i. Pyogenic (most common)

         ii. Amebic (10%)

         iii. Fungal (10%)

       b. Pathophysiology of pyogenic abscess

         i. Acute cholecystitis

         ii. Ascending cholangitis

TABLE 14.1 — Liver Failure Compared With Normal Function

Normal Function	Liver Failure Manifestation
Uptake and secretion of bile	Jaundice
Production of clotting factors	Coagulopathy
Synthesis of albumin	Hypoalbuminemia (contributes to ascites formation)
Detoxification of portal blood	Encephalopathy

   iii. Gangrenous appendicitis
   iv. Diverticulitis
   v. Gastroduodenal perforations
   vi. Blunt liver trauma
  c. Microbiology
   i. *Escherichia coli, Klebsiella, Enterococcus, Pseudomonas, Bacteriodes fragilis*
  d. Clinical presentation
   i. History
    (1) Inciting event or ongoing condition listed above
    (2) Fevers, chills
    (3) Abdominal pain
    (4) Weight loss
   ii. Physical examination
    (1) Abdominal tenderness (RUQ)
    (2) Jaundice (50%)
    (3) Hepatomegaly (30%)
  e. Laboratory
   i. Leukocytosis
   ii. Elevated liver function test (LFT) results
  f. Imaging
   i. Ultrasound
   ii. Computed tomography (CT) scan
    (1) Cystic lesion with an enhancing (bright) rim; may contain air
  g. Treatment
   i. Broad-spectrum antibiotics (may be sufficient for small abscesses)
   ii. Percutaneous drainage
   iii. Operative drainage
  h. Prognosis
   i. Lethal if untreated
   ii. 15%–25% mortality
   iii. Decreased morbidity with percutaneous drainage
2. Benign liver lesions
  a. Hepatic cysts
   i. Simple cyst (most common)
    (1) Arises from aberrant bile duct during embryonic development

(2) Does not communicate with biliary tree

(3) Solitary in 70% of patients

ii. Clinical presentation

  (1) Often asymptomatic

  (2) Typically symptomatic if larger than 5 cm

iii. Diagnosis

  (1) History

    (A) Nausea, vomiting, abdominal pain

    (B) Early satiety

    (C) Jaundice

  (2) Physical examination

    (A) Abdominal tenderness and mass (rare if small)

iv. Laboratory result

  (1) Normal

v. Imaging

  (1) Ultrasound

    (A) Unilocular anechoic mass

    (B) Density of water

    (C) Smooth margin with a thin wall

  (2) CT scan

    (A) Non-enhancing lesion

    (B) Thin wall

    (C) No septations

vi. Treatment

  (1) Observation if asymptomatic

  (2) Percutaneous drainage

    (A) 100% recurrence and risk of infection—not indicated

  (3) Percutaneous aspiration with sclerotherapy

    (A) Injection of ablating agent (e.g., ethanol)

    (B) Must rule out communication with bile ducts prior to injection

    (C) 10%–20% recurrence

  (4) Operative drainage—most effective

    (A) May be done laparoscopically

    (B) Fenestration (un-roofing)

    (C) Drainage with resection of cyst wall

    (D) No liver parenchyma resection

3. Hepatic adenoma
   a. Occurs in young women taking oral contraceptives (OCPs)
      i. May develop during pregnancy
   b. Clinical presentation
      i. Typically asymptomatic
      ii. May rupture, causing pain, hemorrhage, shock
      iii. Malignant transformation potential
      iv. Risk persists even following lesion disappearance after stopping OCPs
   c. Imaging
      i. CT scan or magnetic resonance imaging (MRI)
   d. Treatment
      i. All lesions proved or suspected to be adenoma should be resected
      ii. Radio-frequency or microwave ablation are evolving
   e. Prognosis
      i. Cure if completely resected
4. Hepatic hemangioma
   a. Etiology and pathogenesis
      i. Most common benign mass of the liver
      ii. Incidence 2%–5% of general population
      iii. Occurs in 5th to 7th decades of life
   b. Clinical presentation
      i. Incidental finding (asymptomatic)—most commonly
      ii. Abdominal pain, distention, early satiety, nausea, vomiting
      iii. Spontaneous rupture (rare)
   c. Differential diagnosis
      i. Adenoma
      ii. Focal nodular hyperplasia
      iii. Regenerative nodule
      iv. Cyst
      v. Primary or metastatic liver tumor
   d. Imaging
      i. Ultrasound
         (1) Uniformly hyperechoic, well-circumscribed mass
      ii. CT scan (four-phase CT: pre-contrast, arterial, venous, washout phases)

(1) Well-defined hypodense lesion on pre-contrast phase

(2) Early intense peripheral enhancement

(3) Progressive central contrast fill-in on delayed images: pathognomonic

  iii. MRI is highly specific, 90% sensitive

(1) Hypointense on T1, hyperintense on T2

(2) Centripetal filling (similar to CT)

(3) Nuclear scan with labeled erythrocytes

(4) Do not biopsy

  e. Treatment

    i. Observation for asymptomatic lesions

    ii. Surgical resection for large, symptomatic, or uncertain lesions

    iii. Enucleation or segmental liver resection

5. Focal nodular hyperplasia (FNH)

  a. Epidemiology

    i. Second most common benign liver tumor

    ii. Prevalent in women in 3rd to 5th decades of life

  b. Etiology

    i. Dysplastic response to vascular malformations

  c. Clinical presentation

    i. Asymptomatic

    ii. No risk of bleeding or malignant transformation

  d. Diagnosis

    i. Clinical findings, laboratory results normal

  e. Imaging

    i. CT scan (four-phase)

(1) Iso- or hypodense in pre-contrast phase

(2) Hyperattenuated in arterial phase with central scarring

(3) Delayed enhancement of central scar

    ii. MRI

  f. Treatment

    i. No therapy for asymptomatic stable lesions

    ii. Embolization

    iii. Segmental resection for symptomatic lesions

6. Hepatocellular carcinoma (HCC)
   a. Epidemiology
      i. Most common primary liver tumor
         (1) Fifth most common cancer worldwide
      ii. Risk factors for HCC
         (1) Cirrhosis
         (2) 90% of HCC patients have cirrhosis
         (3) Hepatitis B and/or C
         (4) Alpha$_1$-antitrypsin deficiency
         (5) Oral contraceptives
   b. Clinical presentation
      i. Usually in setting of viral hepatitis, alcohol or drug abuse, metabolic disorders
      ii. History
         (1) Abdominal pain, nausea, anorexia, weight loss
      iii. Physical examination
         (1) May be normal
         (2) Abdominal distention (ascites)
         (3) Jaundice
         (4) Hepatosplenomegaly
         (5) Spider angiomata, caput medusa
   c. Diagnosis
      i. Elevated liver enzymes and LFT
      ii. Elevated alpha-fetoprotein
      iii. Biopsy controversial
   d. Imaging
      i. CT scan
         (1) Hyperattenuating mass
      ii. MRI (superior to CT)
   e. Treatment
      i. Varies with staging/resectability, patient status, function of uninvolved liver
      ii. Medical management
         (1) Chemotherapy
            (A) Alternative to surgery for poor candidates
            (B) Palliation only
            (C) Adjuvant therapy not effective

iii. Ablative techniques
    (1) Radio-frequency ablation
    (2) Cryoablation
    (3) Percutaneous ethanol injections
    (4) Microwave thermotherapy
iv. Surgical management
    (1) Segmental resections
    (2) Liver transplantation
f. Prognosis
  i. Ablative therapies
    (1) Median survival: 12–18 months
  ii. Chemotherapy (alone)
    (1) Median survival: 6–12 months
  iii. Surgery (for resectable lesions)
    (1) Median survival: 30–40 months
    (2) 5-year survival: 30%–40%

II. GB

A. Anatomy (Table 14.2)
  1. Pear-shaped hollow organ
    a. Fundus, body, infundibulum (Hartmann pouch), neck
  2. Located in gallbladder fossa on visceral surface of liver
    a. Junction between right lobe and median segment of left lobe
  3. Hepatic surface attached to liver by connective tissue
  4. Fundus and nonhepatic surface covered by peritoneum
  5. Cystic duct
    a. Connects GB to bile ducts

TABLE 14.2

Biliary Tree Terminology

Term	Definition
Cholecyst- (prefix)	Gallbladder
Cholecystitis	Inflammation or infection of gallbladder
Cholangio- (prefix)	Bile duct
Cholangiogram	X-ray of bile duct
Cholangitis	Inflammation or infection within bile duct
Cholelithiasis	Stones in biliary tree

    b. Point of cystic duct insertion separates common hepatic from common bile ducts

    c. Normally, 3 mm in diameter and 3–4 cm long

    d. Together with inferior edge of liver and common hepatic duct, forms triangle of Calot (contains the cystic artery) (Fig. 14.1)

B. Physiology

    1. Stores and concentrates bile

    2. Bile secreted in response to fatty meals

        a. 600 mL daily

        b. Mediated by cholecystokinin (CCK)

        c. 50%–70% of bile ejected in 30 minutes

    3. Bile reabsorbed in terminal ileum (entero-hepatic circulation)

C. Pathophysiology (Table 14.3)

    1. Cholelithiasis (gallstones)

        a. Failure to maintain biliary solutes (cholesterol and calcium salts) in a solubilized state

    2. Sludge

        a. Mixture of cholesterol crystals, calcium bilirubinate granules, mucin gel

        b. Pathophysiology similar to that of gallstones

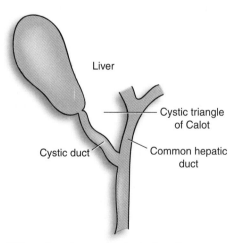

FIGURE 14.1 Biliary ductal anatomy including Calot triangle.

TABLE **14.3**

Clinical Problems Caused by Gallstones According to Position

Position of Gallstone	Clinical Problem
Transient impaction in cystic duct	Biliary colic (RUQ pain)
Permanent impaction in cystic duct	Acute cholecystitis (may progress to hydrops of the gallbladder)
Impaction in common bile duct	Jaundice, cholangitis, or gallstone pancreatitis
Impaction at ampulla of Vater	Jaundice, cholangitis, or gallstone pancreatitis

    c. Classification of gallstones
      i. Cholesterol (75%)
        ii. Black pigment (20%)
        iii. Brown pigment (5%)
  3. Epidemiology
    a. 30% of population in Western world have cholelithiasis
      i. Increased incidence with age
      ii. 70% remain asymptomatic
    b. Risk factors: "F"s: fat, forty, fertile, female
    c. Complications of gallstones
      i. Mildly symptomatic: 1%–3% per year
      ii. Moderately/severely symptomatic: 70% within 1 year
    d. GB disease spectrum
      i. Asymptomatic cholelithiasis

 Asymptomatic gallstones do not require cholecystectomy.

      ii. Symptomatic cholelithiasis
        (1) Biliary colic
        (2) Chronic cholecystitis
        (3) Acute cholecystitis
      iii. Choledocholithiasis
      iv. Cholangitis

v. Gallstone pancreatitis

vi. Gallstone ileus

4. Clinical presentation

  a. Biliary colic

    i. Pathophysiology

      (1) Cystic duct obstruction by a stone

      (2) GB contractions induce pain

    ii. Clinical presentation

      (1) RUQ pain with radiation to right upper back

        (A) Typical onset at 30–45 minutes after meals

        (B) Lasts up to 6 hours

      (2) Nausea/vomiting

      (3) No fevers/chills

      (4) Very mildly tender abdomen

      (5) Normal laboratory test results

      (6) Normal imaging (except gallstones)

    iii. Treatment

      (1) Supportive (pain control)

      (2) Elective cholecystectomy

  b. Chronic cholecystitis

    i. Recurrent attacks of biliary colic

    ii. Mild-to-moderate persistent pain

    iii. Contracted GB on imaging

    iv. Treatment

      (1) Elective cholecystectomy

  c. Acute cholecystitis

    i. Pathophysiology

      (1) Persistent acute cystic duct obstruction

      (2) GB distention due to ongoing mucin production by GB epithelium

      (3) GB wall edema with lymphatic congestion and venous outflow obstruction

      (4) GB necrosis due to resultant arterial insufficiency and hypoperfusion

      (5) Superinfection by dormant bacteria

    ii. Clinical presentation

      (1) RUQ pain (often following fatty/spicy meal)

      (2) Nausea/vomiting

(3) Fevers/chills

(4) Murphy sign

    (A) Arrest of inspiration on deep palpation of RUQ

 In acute cholecystitis, the Murphy sign may be elicited. With the examining hand pressing the RUQ, the patient is asked to take a deep breath. The descending diaphragm pushes the liver and GB to the examiner's hand, eliciting pain (which on examination is known as tenderness) and arrest of inspiration.

    (5) Palpable mass (rare)

iii. Differential diagnosis

    (1) Biliary colic

    (2) Regional enteritis

    (3) Cholangitis

    (4) Pancreatitis

    (5) Bowel obstruction

    (6) Hepatitis

    (7) Urinary tract infection

    (8) Acute myocardial infarction

    (9) Right heart failure

iv. Laboratory findings

    (1) Increased white blood cell (WBC) count

    (2) Elevated LFTs
Alkaline phosphatase, aspartate aminotransferase/alanine aminotransferase (AST/ALT)

    (3) No significant total bilirubin elevation

v. Microbiology

    (1) Positive bile cultures in 50%–75% of patients

    (2) Microorganisms

        (A) *E. coli*

        (B) *Klebsiella*

        (C) *Enterobacter*

        (D) *Proteus*

        (E) *Enterococcus*

      (F) *Pseudomonas*

      (G) *B. fragilis*

  vi. Imaging

    (1) Ultrasound

      (A) Stones (sludge)

      (B) GB wall thickening (more than 3–4 mm)

      (C) Pericholecystic fluid

      (D) Sonographic Murphy sign

    (2) Hepatobiliary iminodiacetic acid (HIDA) scan

      (A) Intravenous (IV) injection of technetium

      (B) Observation of bile movement from liver to duodenum

      (C) No visualization of GB consistent with cystic duct obstruction

      (D) Beware of false-positives

        (i) Liver disease with failure of absorption

        (ii) Distended, bile-filled GB may not fill

        (iii) Seen in patients taking nothing orally (NPO)

  vii. Treatment

    (1) Hospital admission for IV antibiotics, IV fluids, and bowel rest

    (2) Medical therapy, stone dissolution, shock therapy

      (A) Dismal results with high recurrence rates

    (3) Surgery

      (A) Cholecystectomy with or without delay

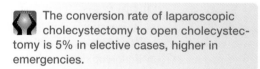

The conversion rate of laparoscopic cholecystectomy to open cholecystectomy is 5% in elective cases, higher in emergencies.

5. Choledocholithiasis

  a. Stone present in the common hepatic/bile ducts

6. Acute cholangitis

  a. Etiology

    i. Infection of the biliary tree

    ii. Choledocholithiasis is the most common etiology

b. Clinical presentation

> The Charcot triad is jaundice, fever, and RUQ pain, which is considered pathognomonic for cholangitis. Untreated, septic shock may ensue, causing hypotension and confusion. With the Charcot triad, this syndrome is known as the Reynold pentad.

  i. Charcot triad
     (1) RUQ pain
     (2) Fever
     (3) Jaundice
  ii. Reynold pentad
     (1) Charcot triad
     (2) Hypotension
     (3) Mental status changes
c. Laboratory findings
  i. Elevated WBC count
  ii. Elevated total bilirubin (>3 mg/dL)
  iii. Elevated direct bilirubin fraction
  iv. Significantly elevated transaminases (AST/ALT)
d. Diagnostic imaging
  i. Ultrasound
     (1) Choledocholithiasis
     (2) Dilated common bile duct (>8 mm)
     (3) Dilated intrahepatic ducts
  ii. Magnetic resonance cholangiopancreatography (MRCP)
     (1) Demonstrates choledocholithiasis
        (A) More sensitive than ultrasound
     (2) Endoscopic ultrasound
        (A) Evolving technique
e. Treatment
  i. Consider intensive care unit (ICU) setting
  ii. Intravenous fluids
  iii. Intravenous antibiotics (after blood cultures are obtained)
  iv. Bowel rest
  v. Early bile duct decompression

        (1) Percutaneous transhepatic cholangiography (PTC)

           (A) Requires dilated intrahepatic biliary system

        (2) Endoscopic retrograde pancreatography (ERCP)

           (A) Gold standard for diagnosis/management of bile duct pathology

           (B) Stone retrieval (90% success rate)

           (C) Sphincterotomy

           (D) Stenting

     vi. Operative bile duct exploration

        (1) If PTC and/or ERCP unsuccessful to decompress duct

7. Gallstone pancreatitis

  a. Leading cause of acute pancreatitis in North America

  b. Pathogenesis

     i. Nonbacterial inflammation of pancreas

     ii. Obstruction of ampulla of Vater by a gallstone

     iii. May occur in setting of only transient choledocholithiasis

  c. Clinical presentation

     i. Epigastric pain with radiation to the back

     ii. Nausea, vomiting

     iii. Anorexia

     iv. Fevers

     v. Abdominal tenderness

     vi. May present with Charcot triad or Reynold pentad

  d. Laboratory findings

     i. Elevated amylase and lipase

     ii. Elevated WBC count

     iii. Elevated bilirubin level (mild)

     iv. Elevated transaminases (ALT >AST)

  e. Diagnostic imaging

     i. Ultrasound

        (1) Confirms cholelithiasis and/or choledocholithiasis

        (2) May demonstrate peripancreatic edema

     ii. CT scan

        (1) Best used to assess anatomic severity of the disease

        (2) May be normal

  f. Treatment

     i. Mild disease

        (1) Bowel rest, IV fluids

(2) Resolution of symptoms in 70%–80% patients within 48 hours

(3) Prophylactic cholecystectomy with an intraoperative cholangiogram before discharge

ii. Severe disease

(1) Bowel rest, IV fluids, antibiotics

(2) ERCP/sphincterotomy in the setting of ongoing ductal obstruction or worsening clinical picture

(3) Operative decompression if ERCP is unsuccessful

iii. Cholecystectomy prior to discharge (if/when medically stable)

iv. ERCP/sphincterotomy may be sufficient in poor surgical candidates to prevent future biliary complications

8. Biliary dyskinesia

　a. Primary motility GB disorder

　　i. Failure of the GB as a pump

　　ii. Symptoms are similar to gallstone disease

　　　(1) Postprandial pain predominant

　　iii. Diagnosis by hepatobiliary iminodiacetic acid (HIDA) scan with cholecystokinin (CCK) injection

　　　(1) Ejection fraction of <35% is diagnostic

　　iv. Treatment: cholecystectomy

9. Gallstone ileus

　a. Form of a small-bowel obstruction (SBO)

　b. Typical signs and symptoms of an SBO

　c. Etiology

　　i. Erosion of large gallstone through gallbladder wall into duodenum

　　ii. Occurs in setting of chronic cholecystitis

　　iii. Elderly/debilitated patient

　　iv. Stone lodges at ileocecal valve, creating bowel obstruction

　　v. Stone seen on abdominal x-ray or CT scan

　d. Treatment

　　i. Emergent exploration

　　ii. Removal of gallstone via small-bowel enterotomy

　　iii. No bowel resection

　　iv. Cholecystectomy

10. Gallbladder carcinoma
  a. Epidemiology
      i. Most common biliary malignancy
      ii. 1.2 cases per 100,000 persons per year
  b. Etiology
      i. GB disease
      ii. Large gallstones (unclear association)
      iii. Female sex
      iv. Multiparity
      v. Obesity
  c. Clinical presentation
      i. May be asymptomatic
      ii. RUQ pain
      iii. Nausea, vomiting, anorexia
      iv. Advanced disease
  d. Weight loss, fatigue, jaundice, firm mass, duodenal obstruction
  e. Diagnostic imaging
      i. Ultrasound or CT scan
          (1) Calcified GB wall
          (2) Discontinuous wall layer
          (3) Large mass (larger than 1 cm)
          (4) Loss of interface between GB and liver
          (5) Lymphadenopathy
  f. Laboratory findings
      i. Elevated alkaline phosphatase
      ii. Elevate bilirubin level
      iii. Elevated gamma-glutamyltransferase (GGT)
      iv. Elevated carcinoembryonic antigen (CEA) and carbohydrate antigen (CA) 19-9
  g. Treatment
      i. Cholecystectomy
          (1) No need for reoperations for incidentally discovered stage 1 tumors
      ii. Cholecystectomy with lymphadenectomy
          (1) If known/suspected preoperatively
              (A) Avoid laparoscopy
          (2) May be sufficient for small (stage 1) tumors

iii. Radical cholecystectomy (with resection of the liver
   bed) for larger tumors
   (1) Partial (non-anatomic) hepatectomy
   (2) Segmental hepatic resection
iv. Adjuvant chemotherapy
v. Radiation therapy
vi. Prognosis extremely poor

MENTOR TIPS DIGEST

- The most common cause of liver failure requiring transplantation in the United States is hepatitis C.
- Asymptomatic gallstones do not require cholecystectomy.
- In acute cholecystitis, the Murphy sign may be elicited. With
  the examining hand pressing the RUQ, the patient is asked to
  take a deep breath. The descending diaphragm pushes the
  liver and GB to the examiner's hand, eliciting pain (which on
  examination is known as tenderness).
- The conversion rate of laparoscopic cholecystectomy to open
  cholecystectomy is 5% in elective cases, higher in emergencies.
- The Charcot triad is jaundice, fever, and RUQ pain, which is
  considered pathognomonic for cholangitis. Untreated, septic
  shock may ensue, causing hypotension and confusion. With
  the Charcot triad, this syndrome is known as Reynold pentad.

Resources

Kitano S, Matsumoto T, Aramaki M, et al. Laparoscopic cholecystectomy
   for acute cholecystitis. Journal of Hepato-Biliary-Pancreatic Surgery
   9:534–537, 2002.
Mansour A, Watson W, Shayani V, et al. Abdominal operations in patients
   with cirrhosis: Still a major surgical challenge. Surgery 122:730, 1997.
Torzilli G, Minagawa M, Takayama T, et al. Accurate preoperative evaluation of liver mass lesions without fine-needle biopsy. Hepatology
   30:889, 1999.

Chapter Self-Test Questions

Circle the correct answer. After you have responded to the questions, check your answers in Appendix A.

1. Which of the following is not part of the portal triad?

    a. Hepatic vein

    b. Hepatic artery

    c. Portal vein

    d. Bile duct

2. What is the treatment of *Echinococcus* liver abscess?

    a. Broad-spectrum antibiotic

    b. Percutaneous drainage and broad-spectrum antibiotic

    c. Albendazole

    d. Surgery and albendazole

3. Which of the following is the most common benign hepatic tumor?

    a. Hepatic adenoma

    b. Hepatic hemangioma

    c. Focal nodular hyperplasia

    d. Liver cyst

4. Which of the following are primary bile salts?

    a. Cholate and lithocholate

    b. Cholate and chenodeoxycholate

    c. Chenodeoxycholate and lithocholate

    d. Lithocholate and deoxycholate

PART

5. A 65-year-old male with diabetes mellitus presents with blood pressure of 80/40, fever, mild RUQ abdominal pain, and mental status change. Laboratory results reveal elevated liver enzyme, normal lipase, and normal WBC count. What is the most likely diagnosis?

a. Acute cholecystitis

b. Cholangitis

c. Necrotizing gallstone pancreatitis

d. Choledocholithiasis

See the testbank CD for more self-test questions.

15

SPLEEN

Yuri W. Novitsky, MD

I. Anatomy

- **A.** Second largest organ of the reticuloendothelial system
  - **1.** Arises from cluster of mesenchymal cells
  - **2.** Non-fusion leads to accessory spleens (15%–30%)
  - **3.** Location (most to least common)
    - **a.** Hilum
    - **b.** Pancreatic tail
    - **c.** Omentum
    - **d.** Splenic artery
    - **e.** Splenocolic ligament
    - **f.** Mesentery
- **B.** Located in posterior left upper quadrant (LUQ)
  - **1.** Convex parietal surface
  - **2.** Concave visceral surface
  - **3.** Covered by peritoneum (except for hilum)
- **C.** Attached to surrounding organs by multiple avascular suspensory ligaments
  - **1.** Splenophrenic (to diaphragm)
  - **2.** Splenorenal (to left kidney)
  - **3.** Splenocolic (to splenic flexure of colon)
    - **a.** Close association with tortuous inferior pole vessels and/or left gastroepiploic artery
  - **4.** Gastrosplenic (to greater curve of stomach)
    - **a.** Contains short gastric vessels
- **D.** Splenic parenchyma
  - **1.** Normal adult size: 12–14 cm in craniocaudal direction
  - **2.** Normal weight: 150–200 g

3. Enveloped by thin (easily injured) capsule

4. Contains red and white pulp

E. Vascular anatomy

  1. Arterial supply

    a. Splenic artery (from celiac trunk)

      i. Splenic vessels traverse abdomen along superior aspect of pancreas

    b. Short gastric arteries (from splenic and left gastroepiploic arteries)

  2. Venous outflow

    a. Splenic vein

      i. Polar veins from splenic hilum

      ii. Tributary to portal vein

II. Splenic Tumors

A. Benign tumors

  1. Hemangioma

    a. Most common primary non-lymphoid tumor

    b. Usually associated with hemangiomas at other sites (liver, intestine)

    c. May rupture spontaneously or after trauma

    d. Splenectomy, if symptomatic/ruptured

  2. Hamartoma

    a. Typically asymptomatic

    b. Solid or cystic mass on abdominal imaging

    c. Splenectomy to establish/confirm diagnosis, rule out malignancy

  3. Lymphangioma

    a. Benign cystic lesion

    b. Associated with other cystic abnormalities (bone, skin, kidney)

    c. Splenectomy to establish/confirm diagnosis, rule out malignancy

B. Malignant tumors

  1. Non-Hodgkin's lymphoma (most common)

    a. Epidemiology

      i. Usually by extension from other sites

      ii. Average patient 50 years old

      iii. B-cell tumor

    b. Presenting features (may be asymptomatic)
       i. Splenomegaly
      ii. Fevers, night sweats, weight loss, fatigue
    c. Diagnosis
       i. Computed tomography (CT)
         (1) May reveal a mass, requiring splenectomy
      ii. Biopsy of enlarged lymph nodes
         (1) May be deferred until splenectomy (if no other nodes involved)
    d. Treatment
       i. Chemotherapy
      ii. Radiation may be added
      iii. Splenectomy
         (1) Symptomatic splenic mass
         (2) Splenomegaly without lymphadenopathy
    e. Prognosis
       i. 80%–90% 5-year survival
      ii. Better prognosis with nodular form
 2. Hodgkin lymphoma
    a. Epidemiology
       i. Bimodal age distribution (late 20s and older than 50 years)
      ii. More common in men
    b. Presenting features
       i. Asymptomatic lymphadenopathy
         (1) Cervical (65%–80%)
         (2) Axillary (10%–15%)
         (3) Inguinal (6%–12%)
         (4) Spleen (10%)
      ii. Constitutional symptoms
         (1) Fevers, night sweats, malaise, lethargy, anorexia, weakness
    c. Diagnosis
       i. CT scan
      ii. Lymph-node biopsy (excisional)
      iii. Splenectomy for staging
         (1) Not commonly performed today
    d. Treatment
       i. Chemoradiation

PART

ii. Splenectomy for symptomatic splenomegaly

e. Prognosis
   i. 85%–90% 5-year survival
   ii. Decreases with higher stage
   iii. 5% 5-year survival if left untreated

3. Angiosarcoma
   a. Most common malignant non-lymphoid splenic neoplasm
   b. Central tumor necrosis on CT scan
   c. Aggressive tumor biology with early metastasis
   d. Spontaneous tumor rupture with intra-abdominal hemorrhage
   e. Treated with splenectomy (typically palliative)
   f. Poor prognosis

III. Splenic Cysts
   A. True (with epithelial lining) and pseudocysts
   1. True nonparasitic cysts
      a. Epidemiology
         i. 20% of all splenic cysts
         ii. Children and young adults
      b. Histology
         i. Epidermoid
         ii. Dermoid
         iii. Neoplastic (benign)
      c. Clinical presentation
         i. Incidental finding
         ii. Rarely symptomatic, unless larger than 8 cm
         iii. Abdominal pain
         iv. Early satiety
         v. Postprandial nausea
      d. Complications
         i. Superinfection
         ii. Spontaneous rupture
         iii. Hemorrhage
      e. Diagnosis
         i. Physical examination (splenomegaly, LUQ mass)
         ii. CT scan
      f. Treatment
         i. Splenectomy

    2. True parasitic cysts
        a. Parasitic (hydatid)—most common worldwide
            i. Echinococcus granulosus
            ii. Usually in setting of hydatid liver disease
            iii. Abdominal pain, fevers, chills
            iv. Splenectomy (avoid cyst rupture)

B. Pseudocyst
    1. Cystic lesion without epithelial lining
    2. Secondary to pancreatitis or splenic trauma
    3. Clinical presentation similar to true nonparasitic cyst
    4. Splenectomy for cysts larger than 8 cm

IV. Splenic Abscess
A. Etiology
    1. Hematogenous spread (most common)
        a. Bacterial endocarditis
        b. Pyelonephritis
        c. Intravenous (IV) drug abuse
        d. Lung abscess
    2. Secondary superinfection
        a. Splenic trauma/hematoma
        b. Splenic infarction
        c. Sickle cell anemia/crisis
    3. Direct extension
        a. From adjacent intra-abdominal abscess

B. Microbiology
    1. *Staphylococcus*
    2. *Streptococcus*
    3. *Salmonella*
    4. *Escherichia coli*
    5. Anaerobes
    6. Parasites

C. Clinical presentation
    1. Fatigue
    2. Abdominal pain/tenderness
    3. Fevers/chills
    4. Leukocytosis

D. Diagnosis
    1. History and physical examination

    2. CT scan

      a. Low-density non-enhancing lesion

      b. Contains gas and/or air-fluid level

  E. Treatment

    1. Broad-spectrum antibiotics

    2. Percutaneous drainage

    3. Splenectomy

    4. Partial splenectomy (rarely indicated)

V. Splenic Artery Aneurysm

  A. Etiology

    1. Dysplasia of media layer in young females

      a. Propensity for rupture during pregnancy

    2. Atherosclerosis in males

    3. Focal arterial injury

      a. Pancreatitis

      b. Trauma

    4. Arteritis

    5. Portal hypertension

  B. Clinical presentation

    1. Asymptomatic—most

    2. Vague abdominal pain

    3. Postprandial fullness, nausea

    4. Aneurysmal rupture

      a. Bleeding into lesser sac—limited early on

      b. Exsanguinating intraperitoneal rupture—often fatal

  C. Diagnosis

    1. High index of suspicion

    2. Abdominal plain films

      a. "Eggshell" calcification in mid-abdomen

    3. CT scan

  D. Treatment

    1. Aneurysm resection with or without (preferred) splenectomy

    2. Reserved for symptomatic aneurysms or asymptomatic aneurysms in women of childbearing age

    3. Endovascular stenting

VI. Splenectomy

  A. Generalized indications

    1. Trauma

The most common indication for splenectomy is traumatic splenic rupture.

2. Symptomatic splenomegaly
3. Hypersplenism
4. Hematologic abnormalities
   a. Hemolytic anemia
   b. Spherocytosis
   c. Thrombocytopenia
      i. Idiopathic thrombocytopenic purpura (ITP) most common indication for elective splenectomy
5. Splenic masses
6. Diagnostic
   a. Hodgkin disease
B. Preoperative consideration
   1. Immunizations 2 weeks preoperation
   2. Bowel preparation
   3. Platelet transfusion, if needed (in holding area)
   4. Packed red blood cells (RBCs) readily available
   5. Stress-dose steroids, if needed
C. Technique/steps of the operation
   1. Mobilization of spleen via division of suspensory ligaments
      a. Lateral, inferior, superior
   2. Identification/preservation of pancreatic tail
   3. Division of hilar vascular pedicle
   4. Division of short gastric vessels
   5. Identification and removal of accessory spleens
      a. May result in surgical failure if missed
   6. Placement of specimen in retrieval bag (morcellation) and removal
D. Approaches
   1. Open
      a. Established method
      b. Supine position
      c. Midline or right subcostal incision
      d. Most commonly performed for trauma
   2. Laparoscopic
      a. Emerging as gold standard

      b. Right lateral decubitus position (right side down)

      c. Morcellation prior to removal (no large incision needed)

      d. Decreased pain, faster postoperative recovery versus open

   3. Hand-assisted laparoscopic

      a. Reserved for larger spleens

         i. Larger than 22–23 cm in craniocaudal length

         ii. Larger than 18 cm in transverse length

      b. Ease in splenic dissection, manipulation, retrieval

      c. Positioning similar to laparoscopy

      d. Periumbilical midline hand-access incision (6–7 cm)

      e. Postoperative recovery parallels those of pure laparoscopic techniques

E. Postoperative changes

   1. Transient leukocytosis (may stay elevated up to 6 months)

   2. Thrombocytosis (may need antiplatelet therapy)

   3. Howell-Jolly bodies (nuclear fragments of DNA in the RBCs)

   4. Siderocytes (RBCs with iron-containing granules)

F. Perioperative complications

   1. Bleeding

      a. Capsular tears

      b. Poor control or tear from hilar and/or short gastric vessels

   2. Pancreatic injury/leak

      a. Postoperative pain, fevers, leukocytosis

      b. Diagnosed with CT scan

      c. Treated with percutaneous drainage, bowel rest, total parenteral nutrition (TPN), octreotide

   3. Portal/splenic vein thrombosis

      a. 5%–14% of patients

      b. Increased incidence in myeloproliferative disorders, massive splenomegaly

      c. Possible association with postoperative thrombocytopenia

      d. Antiplatelet therapy for platelet counts over 1–1.5 million/mm^3

      e. Clinical presentation (varies)

         i. Symptoms absent or vague

         ii. Abdominal discomfort

         iii. Tenderness

         iv. Fevers/leukocytosis

         v. Signs/symptoms of bowel ischemia/necrosis

            (1) May be catastrophic and fatal

   f. Diagnosis
      i. High index of suspicion
      ii. Abdominal duplex ultrasonography
      iii. CT scan
   g. Treatment
      i. Expectant for asymptomatic patients
      ii. Systemic anticoagulation
      iii. Thrombolytics
      iv. Surgical exploration for compromised bowel
4. Overwhelming postsplenectomy sepsis (OPSS)
   a. Incidence 1%–4%
      i. More common in children
   b. Most commonly occurs during first asplenic year
   c. Microbiology
      i. *Streptococcus pneumoniae*
      ii. *Haemophilus influenzae*
      iii. *Neisseria meningitis*
   d. Vaccination (against encapsulated bacteria)
      i. 2 weeks preoperatively or
      ii. 2 weeks postoperatively

VII. Hematologic Indications for Splenectomy
A. RBC-related indications
1. Hereditary spherocytosis
   a. Pathogenesis
      i. Inherited dysfunction/deficiency of RBC membrane
      protein
        (1) Loss of membrane surface area
        (2) Lack of RBC deformability
        (3) RBC sequestration and destruction by spleen
   b. Clinical presentation
      i. Patients often asymptomatic
      ii. Splenomegaly common
   c. Treatment
      i. Splenectomy (curative in more than 90% of patients)
        (1) Perform concurrent with cholecystectomy
        (pigmented gallstones)
        (2) Delay in children until older than 4 years old to
        avoid OPSS

2. Autoimmune hemolytic anemia
  a. Pathogenesis
    i. RBCs opsonized by antibodies
    ii. Phagocytosis by splenic macrophages or intravascular hemolysis
  b. Clinical presentation
    i. Chronic anemia main feature
    ii. Splenomegaly rare
  c. Treatment
    i. Corticosteroids
    ii. Blood transfusion
    iii. Surgery for failure of medical therapy
  d. Prognosis
    i. 70%–80% with favorable clinical response
3. Sickle cell anemia
  a. Pathogenesis
    i. Mutation in hemoglobin chain
      (1) Changes in RBC shape
      (2) Lack of RBC deformability
      (3) Microvascular congestion by RBCs
  b. Clinical presentation
    i. Sickle cell crisis
    ii. Diffuse pain, tissue ischemia/necrosis
  c. Treatment
    i. Supportive (hydration, pain control)
    ii. Indications for splenectomy (palliation)
      (1) Acute sequestration crisis
      (2) Hypersplenism
      (3) Splenic abscess
4. Thalassemia
  a. Disorder of hemoglobin synthesis
    i. Severe anemia
  b. Treatment
    i. Blood transfusion
    ii. Parenteral chelating agents
  c. Indications for splenectomy
    i. Excessive transfusion requirements
    ii. Painful splenomegaly
    iii. Symptomatic splenic infarction

B. Platelet-related indications
　1. Idiopathic thrombocytic purpura (ITP)
　　a. Pathogenesis
　　　i. Platelet destruction
　　　ii. Child form often self-limiting (ITP/hemolytic uremic syndrome [HUS])
　　b. Clinical presentation

 ITP spleens are normal size.

　　　i. Severe thrombocytopenia
　　　ii. Bleeding complications
　　　iii. Extensive purpura
　　c. Treatment
　　　i. Medical
　　　　(1) Systemic corticosteroids
　　　　(2) Intravenous immunoglobulin
　　　ii. Indications for splenectomy
　　　　(1) Failure of medical therapy
　　　　(2) Intolerance of systemic steroids
　　　　(3) Relapse after cessation of steroid therapy
　　d. Outcomes
　　　i. Medical therapy: 50%–75% resolution
　　　ii. Splenectomy: 70%–90% resolution
　　　　(1) More favorable if good response to prior medical therapy
　2. Thrombocytic thrombocytopenic purpura
　　a. Pathogenesis
　　　i. Enzymatic deficiency (congenital or acquired)
　　　ii. Circulation of large molecules of von Willebrand factor
　　　iii. Platelet clumping
　　　iv. Microvascular thrombotic episodes
　　b. Clinical presentation
　　　i. Malaise, fever, diarrhea
　　　ii. Petechiae, bruising
　　　iii. Neurologic changes

       iv. Transient paralysis

       v. Renal failure

   c. Diagnosis

       i. Clinical; no specific tests

   d. Treatment

       i. Medical

          (1) Plasma exchange

          (2) Plasmapheresis

          (3) Systemic steroids

          (4) Immunosuppression

       ii. Surgical

          (1) Indications for splenectomy

             (A) Failure of medical therapy

             (B) Frequent relapses

          (2) Avoid preoperative platelet transfusions

C. White blood cell–related indications

  1. Leukemia

   a. Chronic lymphocytic leukemia

   b. Hairy cell leukemia

   c. Indications for splenectomy

       i. Severe cytopenia

       ii. Facilitation of chemotherapy

       iii. Symptomatic splenomegaly

  2. Lymphoma

D. Bone marrow–related indications

  1. Myelofibrosis

  2. Myeloproliferative disorders (MPDs)

   a. Chronic myeloid leukemia

   b. Acute myeloid leukemia

   c. Essential thrombocytopenia

   d. Polycythemia vera

  3. Indication for splenectomy

   a. Symptomatic splenomegaly

   b. Increased perioperative morbidity in patients with MPD

MENTOR TIPS DIGEST

- The most common indication for splenectomy is traumatic splenic rupture.
- ITP spleens are normal size.

Resources

Cadili A. Complications of splenectomy. American Journal of Medicine 121:371–375, 2008.

Holterman AXL, et al. Surgical management of pediatric hematologic disorders. Surgical Clinics of North America 86, 2006.

Chapter Self-Test Questions

Circle the correct answer. After you have responded to the questions, check your answers in Appendix A.

1. The most common location of an accessory spleen is the:

   a. Omentum

   b. Splenic artery

   c. Splenic hilum

   d. Mesentery

2. All of the following are peritoneal ligaments that support the spleen *except:*

   a. Coronary ligament

   b. Gastrosplenic ligament

   c. Splenorenal ligament

   d. Phrenocolic ligament

3. All of the following are common indications for splenectomy *except:*

   a. Trauma

   b. Hypersplenism

   c. Hereditary spherocytosis

   d. Sickle cell disease

   e. ITP

4. Patients undergoing splenectomy should be immunized against all of the following organisms *except:*

   a. *S. pneumoniae*

   b. *S. aureus*

   c. *H. influenzae*

   d. *N. meningitides*

5. Patients with the highest risk of OPSS are:

   a. Trauma patients

   b. The pediatric population

   c. Patients who take penicillin for prophylaxis after splenectomy

   d. Patients who receive their vaccinations after splenectomy

See the testbank CD for more self-test questions.

16

PANCREAS

Louis Reines, MD, and Robert Kozol, MD

I. Anatomy

A. Retroperitoneal position

  1. Lies posterior to stomach and lesser omentum

  2. Extends from second portion of duodenum to splenic hilum

   a. 10–20 cm in length

   b. Covered by peritoneum anteriorly

   c. Lies in proximity posteriorly to inferior vena cava (IVC), superior mesenteric vessels, the aorta at L1, and the right renal vein

B. Four portions and vascular distribution

  1. Head and uncinate process

   a. Lies within duodenal C-shaped loop

   b. Includes posteroinferior extension called uncinate process

   c. Superior mesenteric artery (SMA) and superior mesenteric vein (SMV) run posterior to pancreas

   d. Supplied by superior pancreaticoduodenal artery, a branch of gastroduodenal artery, which is a branch of the common hepatic artery, which comes off the celiac axis

   e. Also supplied by inferior pancreaticoduodenal artery, which is a branch of SMA

  2. Neck

   a. Anterior to superior mesenteric and portal veins

   b. Supplied by branches of splenic and left gastroepiploic artery

  3. Body

   a. Lies to left of neck

   b. Supplied by branches of splenic and left gastroepiploic artery (dorsal pancreatic artery)

    4. Tail
        a. In contact with splenic hilum
        b. Supplied by inferior pancreatic artery
  C. Lymphatic drainage
    1. Head
        a. Nodes in pancreaticoduodenal groove communicate with subpyloric, portal, mesocolic, mesenteric, and aortocaval nodes
    2. Body and tail
        a. Drain to retroperitoneal nodes in splenic hilum or to celiac, aortocaval, mesocolic, or mesenteric nodes
  D. Visceral innervation
    1. Sympathetic
        a. Arises from cell bodies in thoracic sympathetic ganglia and transverse celiac ganglia and ends in retroperitoneal tissue
        b. Principal pathway for pancreatic pain
    2. Parasympathetic
        a. Cell bodies originate in vagal nuclei, travel in posterior vagal trunk and transverse celiac plexus, and end in pancreatic parenchyma
        b. Serve exclusively efferent function

II. Pancreatitis

  A. Acute pancreatitis
    1. Pathophysiology
        a. Acute inflammatory process
            i. Ranges from mild parenchymal edema to severe hemorrhagic pancreatitis, leading to necrosis
        b. Intracellular activation of trypsinogen to trypsin leads to activation of other proenzymes and cellular autodigestion
    2. Epidemiology

 The two most common causes of pancreatitis are alcohol abuse and gallstones.

        a. Idiopathic (10%–20%)
        b. Gallstones (40%–60%)
        c. Ethanol (20%–30%)
        d. Trauma
        e. Scorpion bite

    f. Mumps and other viruses

    g. Autoimmune

    h. Steroids

    i. Hyperlipidemia

    j. Post–endoscopic retrograde cholangiopancreatography (ERCP)

    k. Drugs

    l. Hypercalcemia

3. Prevention

    a. Stop drinking

    b. Interval cholecystectomy (33% of patients with recurrence by 8 weeks, if no early cholecystectomy))

4. Symptoms

    a. Epigastric pain

    b. Nausea

    c. Vomiting

    d. Back pain

5. Signs

    a. Epigastric tenderness

    b. Diffuse abdominal tenderness

    c. Adynamic ileus

    d. Fever

    e. Shortness of breath (SOB)

    f. Dehydration

    g. Tachycardia

    h. Shock

    i. Hemorrhage

        i. Grey Turner sign—bluish discoloration of left flank

        ii. Cullen sign—bluish discoloration of periumbilical area

        iii. Fox sign—bluish discoloration below inguinal ligament

    j. Pleural effusion

    k. Disseminated intravascular coagulation (DIC)

6. Differential diagnosis

    a. Gastritis/peptic ulcer disease (PUD)

    b. Perforated viscus

    c. Acute cholecystitis

    d. Small-bowel obstruction (SBO)

    e. Mesenteric ischemia

    f. Ruptured abdominal aortic aneurysm (AAA)

g. Biliary colic

h. Inferior myocardial infarction (MI)

7. Diagnostic findings
    a. Laboratory test results—increased amylase, lipase, white blood cells (WBCs)
    b. Abnormal x-ray (AXR)—sentinel loop (dilated jejunum), colon cutoff
    c. Ultrasound (U/S)—pseudocyst, phlegmon, abscess, cholelithiasis
    d. Computed tomography (CT)—peri-pancreatic inflammation, pseudocyst, phlegmon, abscess, pancreatic necrosis

8. Treatment
    a. Nothing by mouth (NPO)
    b. Intravenous (IV) fluids
    c. Total parenteral nutrition (TPN)
    d. IV antibiotics in the setting of pancreatic necrosis

 H_2 blockers and antibiotics have not been shown to affect the course of acute pancreatitis.

    e. Analgesia
    f. Correction of coagulopathy and electrolytes
    g. Tincture of time
    h. Nasogastric tube (NGT) if vomiting

9. Prognosis
    a. Ranson criteria at presentation
        i. Age older than 55 years
        ii. WBCs more than 16,000
        iii. Glucose levels higher than 200 mg/dL
        iv. Aspartate aminotransferase (AST) higher than 250 IU/L
        v. Lactate dehydrogenase (LDH) level higher than 350 U/L
    b. Ranson criteria at 48 hours
        i. Base deficit >4 (mmol/L bicarbonate)
        ii. Blood urea nitrogen (BUN) increase >5 mg/dL
        iii. Fluid sequestration >6 L
        iv. Hematocrit (Hct) decrease >10%
        v. P_{O_2} <60 mm Hg

   c. Mortality per positive criteria
      i. 0–2, less than 5%
      ii. 3–4, 5%
      iii. 5–6, 40%
      iv. 7–8, 100%
 10. Complications
   a. Pseudocyst
   b. Abscess/infection
   c. Pancreatic necrosis
   d. Splenic/mesenteric/portal vein thrombosis or rupture
   e. Acute respiratory distress syndrome (ARDS)/sepsis/ multiple system organ failure (MSOF)
   f. Coagulopathy/disseminated intravascular coagulation (DIC)
B. Chronic pancreatitis
  1. Pathophysiology
   a. Chronic inflammation
   b. Destruction of parenchyma
   c. Fibrosis and calcification
   d. Destruction of endocrine and exocrine tissue
  2. Epidemiology
   a. Alcohol abuse (70%)
   b. Idiopathic (15%)
   c. Hypercalcemia
   d. Hyperlipidemia
   e. Familial
  3. Signs
   a. Steatorrhea
   b. Diabetes
  4. Symptoms
   a. Unrelenting pain
   b. Recurrent pain
   c. Weight loss
   d. Diarrhea
   e. Diabetes
  5. Differential diagnosis
   a. Peptic ulcer disease (PUD)
   b. Biliary tract disease

      c. Ruptured abdominal aortic aneurysm (AAA)

      d. Pancreatic cancer

      e. Angina

  6. Laboratory tests

      a. Increased or normal amylase/lipase

      b. Increase in 72-hour fecal fat analysis

      c. Failed glucose tolerance test

  7. Diagnostic findings

      a. Triple-phase CT scan: atrophy, diffuse calcifications, dilated pancreatic ducts

      b. ERCP/magnetic resonance cholangiopancreatography (MRCP): ductal irregularities with alternating stenosis and dilation, giving "chain of lakes" appearance, pseudocysts

      c. AXR: pancreatic calcification

  8. Medical treatment

      a. Discontinuation of alcohol use

      b. Insulin for diabetes mellitus (DM)

      c. Pancreatic enzyme replacement

      d. Narcotics for pain

      e. Low-fat diet

      f. Octreotide may decrease pain

  9. Surgical treatment (for pain relief)

      a. Near total pancreatectomy (if no dilated ducts)

      b. Puestow—longitudinal pancreaticojejunostomy for ductal dilation

      c. Berger—duodenum-preserving resection of pancreatic head combined with Roux-en-Y drainage of retained main pancreatic duct in neck of the gland

      d. Frey—side-to-side pancreaticojejunostomy with anterior central resection of pancreatic head

C. Complications of acute pancreatitis

  1. Pseudocyst

      a. Encapsulated collection of pancreatic fluid that persists more than 4 weeks

      b. Result of walling off pancreatic duct disruption

      c. Contains high concentration of enzymes, including amylase, lipase, trypsin

      d. Develops in 10% of patients after attack of acute alcoholic pancreatitis

e. Most commonly caused by chronic pancreatitis
f. Symptoms
  i. Epigastric pain
  ii. Emesis
  iii. Fever
  iv. Persistent pain past acute episode of pancreatitis
  v. Weight loss
g. Signs
  i. Palpable epigastric mass
  ii. Tender epigastrium
  iii. Ileus
h. Diagnostic findings
  i. Laboratory test results—high amylase, WBC count
  ii. U/S—fluid-filled mass
  iii. CT—fluid-filled mass
  iv. ERCP—radiopaque contrast material–filled cyst
i. Differential diagnosis
  i. Cystadenocarcinoma
  ii. Cystadenoma
j. Treatment
  i. Must wait 6 weeks between start of episode of pancreatitis and elective operative intervention to allow satisfactory internal drainage and maturity of wall
  ii. Pseudocysts larger than 5 cm have a small chance of resolving and higher chance of complication
  iii. Pseudocyst adherent to stomach—cystogastrostomy
  iv. Pseudocyst adherent to duodenum—cystoduodenostomy
  v. Pseudocyst in pancreatic tail—distal pancreatectomy with pseudocystectomy
  vi. Must biopsy cyst wall to rule out malignancy when doing operative procedure
k. Complications
  i. Bleeding
  ii. Infection
  iii. Pancreatic ascites
  iv. Fistula
  v. Gastric outlet obstruction

2. External pancreatic fistula
   a. Drainage of pancreatic exocrine secretion through abdominal wound that persists for more than 7 days
   b. High-output fistula—drains more than 200 mL/day
   c. Low-output fistula—drains less than 200 mL/day
   d. Complications include sepsis, electrolyte abnormalities, skin excoriation
   e. Fistulas in tail managed with distal pancreatectomy
   f. Fistulas in head, neck, or body managed by Roux-en-Y pancreaticojejunostomy
3. Pancreatic abscess
   a. Infected peripancreatic purulent fluid collection
   b. Signs/symptoms
      i. Fever
      ii. Unresolving pancreatitis
      iii. Epigastric mass
   c. Diagnostic tests—CT scan with needle aspiration
   d. Laboratory findings—positive Gram stain and culture
   e. Organisms found—*Escherichia coli, Pseudomonas, Klebsiella, Staphylococcus aureus, Candida*
   f. Treatment—antibiotics and percutaneous drain; operative débridement and drain placement
4. Pancreatic necrosis
   a. Dead pancreatic tissue during episode of acute pancreatitis
   b. Diagnosis—non-enhancement of pancreatic tissue on triple-phase contrast CT scan
   c. Treatment—surgical débridement and drain placement for infected necrosis (based on needle aspiration) or if patient severely ill and refractory to medical management

III. Pancreatic Cancer
A. Epidemiology and risk factors
   1. Six genetic syndromes
      a. Hereditary nonpolyposis colorectal cancer (HNPCC)
      b. Breast cancer type 2 (BRCA2)
      c. Peutz-Jeghers syndrome
      d. Familial atypical multiple mole melanoma (FAMMM)
      e. Hereditary pancreatitis
      f. Ataxia-telangiectasia

   2. Smoking
   3. DM
   4. Chronic pancreatitis
   5. Chemists and coal gas workers
   6. Male-to-female gender ratio 3:2
   7. African-American to white ratio 2:1
   8. Average age older than 60 years
   9. *Rb/p16, p53, DPC4* most often tumor suppressor genes inacti-
      vated in sporadic pancreatic cancer
B. Pathologic features
   1. Duct cell adenocarcinomas (90%)
   2. Adenosquamous carcinoma
   3. Acinar cell carcinoma
   4. 66% arise in head, 33% in body and tail
C. Symptoms

 More than 50% of patients with pancreatic cancer present with abdominal pain and weight loss.

   1. Jaundice
   2. Weight loss
   3. Abdominal pain
   4. Pruritus
D. Physical examination
   1. Palpable gallbladder—Courvoisier sign (due to malignant
      common duct obstruction)
   2. Left supraclavicular adenopathy (Virchow node)
   3. Periumbilical adenopathy (Sister Mary Joseph node)
   4. Drop metastases in pelvis (Blumer shelf)
E. Laboratory findings
   1. Increased direct bilirubin and alkaline phosphatase
   2. Increased liver function tests (LFTs)
   3. Increased carcinoembryonic antigen (CEA) and cancer antigen
      19-9 (CA 19-9)
F. Radiologic findings
   1. Abdominal and pelvic CT scan with IV/oral contrast
      a. Evaluate major blood vessels (look for lack of tumor
         invasion)

    b. Evaluate tumor spread to peripancreatic lymph nodes

    c. Evaluate spread to liver

  2. Magnetic resonance imaging (MRI)/magnetic resonance angiogram (MRA)/MRCP

  3. ERCP

    a. Reserved for cases of obstructive jaundice, but no mass on CT

    b. Chronic pancreatitis and suspicion of pancreatic cancer

G. Pancreatic cancer stages

  1. Stage I—tumor limited to pancreas, no nodes, no metastases

  2. Stage II—tumor extends into bile duct, peripancreatic tissues, or duodenum; no nodes, no metastases

  3. Stage III—same findings as stage II plus positive nodes

  4. Stage IVa—tumor extends to stomach, colon, spleen, with any nodal status, and no metastases

  5. Stage IVb—distant metastases

H. Treatment

  1. Head of pancreas—Whipple procedure (pancreaticoduodenectomy)

    a. Cholecystectomy

    b. Antrectomy

    c. Pancreaticoduodenectomy

    d. Choledochojejunostomy

    e. Pancreaticojejunostomy

    f. Gastrojejunostomy

  2. Complication rate: 30%–40%

    a. Delayed gastric emptying if antrectomy performed

    b. Pancreatic fistula

    c. Intra-abdominal abscess

    d. Wound infection

    e. Metabolic diabetes and pancreatic exocrine insufficiency

  3. Mortality rate: 3%

  4. Body or tail: distal pancreatectomy

 Most patients with pancreatic carcinoma are inoperable for cure.

I. Factors signifying inoperability
   1. Encasement of SMA, SMV, or portal vein
   2. Liver metastases
   3. Peritoneal implants
   4. Distant lymph-node metastases
   5. Distant metastases
      a. Liver (up to 80%)
      b. Peritoneum (60%)
      c. Lungs and pleura (50%–75%)
      d. Adrenal glands (25%)
J. Palliative treatment
   1. Percutaneous transhepatic cholangiograph (PTC)
   2. ERCP and stent placement
K. Prognosis
   1. 90% mortality at 1 year post diagnosis
   2. 5-year survival after resection: 20%

MENTOR TIPS DIGEST

- The two most common causes of pancreatitis are alcohol abuse and gallstones.
- H_2 blockers and antibiotics have not been shown to affect the course of acute pancreatitis.
- More than 50% of patients with pancreatic cancer present with abdominal pain and weight loss.
- Most patients with pancreatic carcinoma are inoperable for cure.

Resources

Carroll JK. Acute pancreatitis: Diagnosis, prognosis, and treatment. American Family Physician 75:1513–1520, 2007.

Elfar M. The inflammatory cascade in acute pancreatitis: Relevance to clinical disease. Surgical Clinics of North America 8:1325–1340, 2007.

Frey CF. Surgery for chronic pancreatitis. American Journal of Surgery. 194:S53–S60, 2007.

Nathens AB. Management of the critically ill patient with severe acute pancreatitis. Critical Care Medicine 32: 2524–2536, 2004.

Townsend CM. Sabiston textbook of surgery, 18th ed. Elsevier, 2007.

Chapter Self-Test Questions

Circle the correct answer. After you have responded to the questions, check your answers in Appendix A.

1. The pancreas receives arterial blood from the:

    a. Superior pancreaticoduodenal artery, which is a branch off the superior mesenteric artery

    b. Superior pancreaticoduodenal artery, which is a branch off the inferior mesenteric artery

    c. Inferior pancreaticoduodenal artery, which is a branch off the superior mesenteric artery

    d. Inferior pancreaticoduodenal artery, which is a branch off the gastro-duodenal artery

2. The two most common causes of acute pancreatitis in the United States are:

    a. Scorpion bites and gallstones

    b. Hyperlipidemia and gallstones

    c. Ethanol and hyperlipidemia

    d. Ethanol and gallstones

3. Grey Turner sign, which can be seen in hemorrhagic pancreatitis, is described as:

    a. Periorbital bruising

    b. Bruising of the flank

    c. Bruising of the area around the umbilicus

    d. Infra-inguinal bruising

4. Initial treatment for acute pancreatitis includes all of the following *except:*

    a. Broad-spectrum antibiotics

    b. Bowel rest (NPO status)

    c. IVF resuscitation

    d. Pain control

    e. NGT if significant vomiting

5. Ranson criteria at presentation include all of the following *except:*

   a. Age

   b. Amylase

   c. WBCs

   d. Glucose

   e. AST

See the testbank CD for more self-test questions.

17

SMALL BOWEL

Mun Jye Poi, MD, and Yuri W. Novitsky, MD

I. Anatomy

  A. Overview

    1. Longest organ in body (15–20 feet)

      a. Duodenal bulb to ileocecal (IC) valve

    2. Duodenum (see Chapter 13)

    3. Jejunum and ileum

      a. Extend from ligament of Treitz (LT) to IC valve

        i. Jejunum

          (1) First 3/5th of small bowel (SB)

          (2) Thicker wall due to thick mucosa

          (3) Lining (prominent plica circulares)

          (4) Wider diameter

        ii. Ileum

          (1) Narrow, especially at IC valve

      b. Invested in mesentery

        i. Mesentery suspends intestine from posterior abdominal wall

        ii. Site of lymphovascular channels

        iii. Base (root) of mesentery about 15 cm

          (1) Extends from LT (to left of L2 body) toward right sacroiliac joint

          (2) 20–25 cm from root to bowel border

  B. Layers of wall

    1. Serosa

      a. Mesothelial cells of visceral peritoneum

    2. Muscularis

      a. Outer longitudinal and inner circular muscles

      b. Myenteric (Auerbach) plexus in between

3. Submucosa
   a. Strongest due to dense connective tissue
   b. Rich network of nerves and lymphovascular channels
   c. Meissner nerve plexus
4. Mucosa
   a. Layers of epithelial cells, connective tissue, and smooth muscle
   b. Contains crypts and villi
C. Blood supply and drainage
   1. Arterial supply
      a. Superior mesenteric artery (SMA) (from aorta)
      b. First jejunal branch
      c. Intestinal branches that form arcades
         i. Vasa recta from peripheral arcades
            (1) Run directly (without cross-communication) to intestinal borders
            (2) Straight and long in jejunum
            (3) Short and arborous in ileum
         ii. Best blood supply at mesenteric and poorest supply at antimesenteric side
   2. Venous drainage parallels arteries
      a. Toward portal vein via superior mesenteric vein
   3. Lymphatics parallel vascular channels
      a. Three sets of lymph nodes
         i. At bowel wall, at arcades, and along SMA
D. Implications for surgery
   1. Small intestine is midline organ
      a. Easiest externalized via midline incision
   2. No clear directionality of any loops
      a. Must palpate ("run") bowel to landmarks (ligament of Treitz and/or IC valve)
   3. Residual length (not resected length) more critical
      a. No need for large resection margins
      b. Preserve IC valve if possible
   4. Distal terminal ileum narrow
      a. Avoid anastomosis near IC valve due to high likelihood of stricture

5. Submucosal layer strongest
   a. Must be included in anastomosis because it would hold the stitches best
6. No collateral circulation at surface of intestine
   a. Do not undercut mesentery close to mesenteric border
   b. Ischemic perforations more likely at antimesenteric side

II. Small-Bowel Obstruction

A. Most common causes of SB obstruction are adhesions and incarcerated inguinal hernias.
   1. Postoperative adhesions: 65%–75% (most common cause)
      a. 20%: within 30 days postoperatively
      b. 30%: within 1 year
      c. 25%: within 5 years
      d. 25%: beyond 5 years
   2. Hernia
      a. Inguinal, femoral, ventral, or internal
   3. Tumors
      a. Primary
      b. Metastatic
   4. Inflammatory bowel disease
   5. Radiation fibrosis
   6. Intussusception (rare in adults)

B. Pathophysiology
   1. Mechanical obstruction of lumen
      a. Extraluminal pressure/"kinking" (adhesions, hernia incarceration)
      b. Intraluminal disorder
   2. Resultant luminal distention
      a. Increased intraluminal pressure
      b. Changes in flow dynamics of bowel wall
         i. Lymphatic flow obstruction
         ii. Venous congestion
         iii. Arterial insufficiency
            (1) Bowel necrosis/perforation

C. Clinical presentation
   1. Varies from subtle discomfort to frank peritonitis
   2. Clinical spectrum
      a. Complete bowel obstruction

b. Closed loop obstruction
3. Partial bowel obstruction
    a. High-grade
    b. Low-grade
D. History
    1. Nausea
    2. Emesis
        a. Non-bloody, bilious, or feculent
    3. Abdominal pain
        a. Insidious onset
        b. Colicky and intermittent
            i. May progress to constant and sharp
        c. Diffuse mid-abdominal
            i. May eventually localize
        d. Typically without radiation
    4. Bowel function
        a. Obstipation (no passage of flatus) for at least 24–48 hours
        b. Constipation (may have bowel movement within first 24 hours)
E. Physical examination
    1. Vital signs
        a. Fever, tachycardia (may not be present early)
    2. Abdominal examination
        a. Distention
            i. May be minimal in proximal or closed-loop obstructions
        b. Diffuse tenderness
            i. May eventually localize late in presentation
        c. Tympany
        d. High-pitch bowel sounds (absent in latter stages)
        e. Empty rectal vault on digital examination
    3. Hernias
        a. Tender, firm mass
        b. May have associated skin changes (severe form)
        c. Critical to inspect whole abdominal wall and both groins
F. Laboratory data
    1. May be normal
    2. Leukocytosis/bandemia
    3. Hypokalemic metabolic alkalosis due to vomiting/dehydration

4. Elevated serum creatinine and blood urea nitrogen (BUN)/ creatinine ratio due to dehydration

5. Metabolic (lactic) acidosis due to bowel ischemia

G. Imaging

    1. Plain abdominal films (obstructive series): initial study of choice

        a. Flat abdomen, upright abdomen, upright chest x-rays

        b. Findings

            i. Distended SB

            ii. Paucity (absence) of distal (large bowel, rectum) air

            iii. Air-fluid levels

            iv. "Thumbprinting": thickened SB wall

            v. Visible plica circulares

            vi. 80% of patients with preceding findings require operation

    2. Computed tomography (CT): increasing in popularity

        a. Sensitivity and specificity above 90%

        b. Both intravenous (IV) and oral contrast

            i. Intraluminal fluid may serve as natural contrast

            ii. Presence of oral contrast in colon and rectum rules out complete SB obstruction

        c. Timing

            i. Initially to confirm/establish diagnosis

            ii. After 24 hours, if no clinical improvement

        d. Findings

            i. Distended proximal bowel

            ii. "Transition zone"

                (1) Border between distended and collapsed bowel

                (2) Area of adhesion or intraluminal obstruction

            iii. Edematous loop(s) of bowel

            iv. Free fluid (ominous sign)

            v. Free air (bowel necrosis/perforation)

            vi. Incarcerated hernia

    3. SB contrast series (SB follow-through)

        a. Not indicated initially

        b. May be helpful in partial SB obstruction

        c. May demonstrate strictures, nearly obstructing lesions, hypomotility

H. Management

> "Do not let sun set on a complete SB obstruction." In cases of complete obstruction, resuscitate the patient, and then go to the operating room.

1. Initial
   a. IV fluids
   b. Nasogastric tube decompression
   c. Foley catheter
   d. No antibiotics unless signs of systemic infection
   e. Judicious use of analgesia unless operative exploration planned
   f. Close observation with serial abdominal examinations
2. Operative exploration
   a. Immediate in lieu of prolonged prehospital course, systemic sepsis, or peritonitis
   b. After 12 hours of observation: "Do not let sun set on a complete SB obstruction"
      i. If no return of bowel function
      ii. Persistent/escalating pain and/or tenderness
      iii. Progressive fever, tachycardia
3. Special considerations
   a. Closed-loop obstruction
      i. Unlikely to resolve with conservative measures
      ii. Warrants immediate/urgent exploration
      iii. Often requires bowel resection due to bowel compromise
   b. Partial SB obstruction
      i. Often lacks typical signs/symptoms of SB obstruction
      ii. Important to differentiate between high- (severe) and low-grade obstructions
      iii. Operative exploration if no improvement in 24–48 hours
         (1) May observe for 3–5 days if signs/symptoms mild
            (A) Follow clinically with serial imaging
            (B) Operative exploration if not complete resolution or failed diet trial

    c. Obstruction in a "virgin" abdomen (patient with no prior abdominal operations)

        i. Operative intervention after initial resuscitation/ stabilization

        ii. Treat underlying cause

        iii. Resection of bowel

          (1) Tumors

          (2) Strangulated bowel

          (3) Intussusception

          (4) Obstructing Crohn disease

        iv. Repair of discovered hernia

          (1) Primarily (just sutures)

          (2) With biologic or absorbable mesh

   d. Obstruction in lieu of known intra-abdominal malignancy

        i. 30% with single adhesion

        ii. 40% with recurrent malignancy amenable to resection

        iii. 30% with carcinomatosis or unresectable malignancy

          (1) No intervention

          (2) Entero-enteric bypass

          (3) Palliative enterostomy

          (4) Gastrostomy

I. Operative considerations

  1. Exploratory laparotomy

    a. Generous incision

        i. Extend beyond previous incisions to virgin abdomen

        ii. Use scalpel instead of electrocautery to avoid thermal bowel injuries

    b. Adhesiolysis

        i. Under direct vision

        ii. Metzenbaum scissors

        iii. Avoid blunt dissection

        iv. Repair serosal tear and enterotomies immediately

    c. Bowel inspection/resection

        i. Run whole length of bowel

        ii. Carefully inspect for viability/injuries

        iii. Resect necrosed segments

        iv. Avoid entero-enteric bypass for benign disease

  2. Laparoscopy

    a. Appropriate for select patients only

   b. Contraindications to laparoscopy
      i. Diffuse peritonitis
      ii. Massively dilated, thin-walled SB (more prone to enterotomies)
      iii. Multiple previous laparotomies
   c. Maintain principles of open explorations
3. Closure
   a. Decompress if possible
      i. Carefully "milk" bowel toward duodenum
   b. Place omentum between SB and abdominal wall
   c. Consider placing anti-adhesion barrier
   d. Close fascia and skin in standard fashion

III. SB Tumors
A. Epidemiology
   1. Relatively uncommon
      a. 2% of all gastrointestinal (GI) malignancies
   2. Benign (60%–70%)
      a. Gastrointestinal stromal tumors (GIST)
      b. Adenoma
      c. Lipoma
      d. Hemangioma
      e. Other
   3. Malignant (30%–40%)
      a. Adenocarcinoma
      b. Carcinoid
      c. Lymphoma
      d. GI Stromal tumors
      e. (Mnemonic: ACLS; in decreasing frequency of occurrence)
B. Clinical presentation
   1. Asymptomatic (often)
      a. Discovered incidentally during surgery, on imaging, or at autopsy
   2. Symptomatic (more than 50% present emergently)
      a. Insidious nonspecific symptoms
      b. Intermittent abdominal pain
      c. Weight loss (almost uniform)
      d. Occult or frank GI bleeding

      e. SB obstruction
          i. Intraluminal mass
          ii. Intussusception with a mass as lead point
      f. Perforation

C. Diagnosis
  1. Plain films rarely diagnostic
  2. SB follow-through
     a. May show filling defects
  3. CT
     a. May suggest tumor histology
     b. Defines extraluminal and distant growth
  4. Angiography
     a. May localize actively bleeding mass
  5. Endoscopy
     a. Technically challenging
     b. May be combined with operative exploration (push enteroscopy)
  6. Capsule endoscopy
     a. Newest technique
     b. Allows for intraluminal imaging
     c. Allows for diagnosis but not localization

D. Clinical features
  1. Adenomas
     a. Most commonly in duodenum
     b. May be associated with familial polyposis syndrome
     c. Present with bleeding, obstruction, or jaundice
     d. Variable malignant potential
     e. Resect endoscopically (in duodenum) or via laparotomy
  2. Lipomas
     a. Duodenum/ileum
     b. Resect if symptomatic (intussusception, luminal obstruction)
  3. Hemangiomas
     a. Single or multiple
     b. Occult or acute bleeding
     c. Difficult to diagnose
         i. Tagged red blood cell scan
         ii. Angiography
         iii. Capsule endoscopy
     d. Resect if symptomatic

4. Adenocarcinoma (30%–50% of malignant SB tumors)

  a. Most frequently in duodenum (40%)

  b. Presentation varies by region

    i. Duodenum (periampullary)

      (1) Obstructive jaundice, bleeding, gastric outlet obstruction

    ii. Jejunum/ileum

      (1) Abdominal pain, weight loss, obstruction (partial)

  c. "Apple-core" appearance on contrast studies

  d. Wide resection

    i. Pancreaticoduodenectomy for ampullary lesions

    ii. Bowel resection with wide margins and a large wedge of mesentery for jejunal/ileal lesions

    iii. Right hemicolectomy for terminal ileum lesions

  e. Prognosis

    i. Very poor due to usual late presentation

    ii. 60%–80% survival for completely resected nonmetastatic jejunal/ileal lesions

5. Carcinoid (20%–30% of malignant SB tumors)

  a. Appendix and ileum most common sites

  b. 80% within 2 feet from ileocecal valve

  c. 30% are multicentric

  d. Presentation

    i. Asymptomatic in 70%–80% of cases

      (1) Incidentally discovered in duodenum during endoscopy

    ii. Symptomatic 20%–30% of cases

      (1) Obstruction

      (2) Carcinoid syndrome

        (A) Diarrhea due to 5-HIAA (serotonin) release

        (B) Flushing

        (C) Palpitations

      (3) Crampy nonspecific pain

    iii. Often metastatic on presentation (70%)

      (1) Liver

      (2) Mesenteric lymph nodes

  e. Diagnosis

    i. Requires high index of suspicion

      ii. Often found at exploration

     iii. Urinary 5-HIAA

        (1) 100% sensitive/specific in metastatic disease

        (2) 75% in nonmetastatic disease

     iv. Imaging

        (1) Abdominal CT

        (2) SB follow-through

        (3) Capsule endoscopy

  f. Management

      i. Surgical therapy

        (1) Complete resection and debulking of metastatic disease

          (A) Small ($<$2 cm) lesions amenable to laparoscopy

        (2) Preoperative and intraoperative somatostatin to avoid carcinoid crisis

        (3) Mandatory complete inspection of intestines for synchronous lesions

          (A) Duodenum

            (i) Enucleation for tumors $<$1 cm

            (ii) Segmental resection for tumors 1–2 cm

            (iii) Pancreaticoduodenectomy for tumors $>$2 cm

          (B) Jejunum/ileum

            (i) Complete resection with large wedge of mesentery

          (C) Liver metastasis

            (i) Wedge resection or ablation

            (ii) Large segmental resections should be delayed

            (iii) Somatostatin (symptom control)

      ii. Adjuvant therapy

        (1) Chemotherapy: response rate of 20%–30%

        (2) Radiation: not indicated

  g. Prognosis

      i. Slow-growing

      ii. Median survival

        (1) Resectable metastatic disease: 15 years

        (2) Unresectable/carcinoid syndrome: 3 years

     iii. Overall 5-year survival: 60%

(1) Small, nonmetastatic tumors: 100%
(2) Metastatic tumors
    (A) Limited/no liver metastasis: 40%–60%
    (B) Diffuse metastasis/carcinoid syndrome: 18%

6. Lymphoma (15%–20% of malignant SB tumors)
  a. Ileum (due to high lymphoid tissue content)
  b. Multifocal in 15%
  c. Middle-aged males
  d. Predisposing factors
    i. Crohn disease
    ii. Celiac sprue
    iii. Immunosuppression
    iv. Transplant
    v. Systemic chemotherapy
    vi. Systemic lupus erythematosus (SLE)
    vii. AIDS
  e. Histopathology
    i. Non-Hodgkin B cell
    ii. Intermediate or high-grade cell features
  f. Presentation
    i. Obstruction, perforation, or hemorrhage in 25% of patients
    ii. Abdominal pain
    iii. Fatigue
    iv. Malaise
    v. Weight loss
  g. Diagnosis
    i. CT
      (1) Mass, thickened bowel, mesenteric lymphadenopathy
    ii. SB follow-through
      (1) Mass; thickened mucosa with ulcerations
    iii. Tissue biopsy (percutaneous or operative)
  h. Treatment
    i. Localized disease
      (1) Wide resection with locoregional lymphadenectomy
        (A) Amenable to laparoscopy
      (2) Adjuvant therapy postoperatively
    ii. Diffuse disease
      (1) Multidrug chemotherapy and radiation

(2) Limited role for debulking

i. Prognosis

    i. Overall 5-year survival: 20%–40%

        (1) Completely resected: 80%

        (2) Disseminated disease: very poor

j. Gastrointestinal stromal tumors (10%–20% of malignant SB tumors)

    i. Jejunum/ileum

    ii. Arise from submucosa (interstitial cells of Cajal)

k. Presentation

    i. Asymptomatic/incidentally discovered

    ii. Symptomatic (50%)

        (1) Abdominal mass

        (2) Abdominal pain

        (3) Weight loss

        (4) Obstruction and bleeding with large tumors

l. Diagnosis

    i. CT

        (1) Extraluminal mass with central necrosis

        (2) Calcifications

    ii. SB follow-through

        (1) Extraluminal mass

            (A) May fill with contrast

        (2) Intraluminal (or dumbbell-shaped) mass

m. Treatment

    i. Complete resection with negative margins

    ii. No lymphadenectomy

    iii. Gleevec (tyrosine kinase inhibitor) for unresectable or metastatic disease

n. Prognosis

    i. Metastatic at presentation/surgery = malignant

        (1) Biologic behavior (not histopathology) determines malignant potential

    ii. Malignant risk

        (1) Size (>5 cm) and mitotic index (>5 mitotic figures per 50 high power fields)

        (2) Postoperative Gleevec under investigation

IV. Meckel Diverticulum (MD)

A. Overview

    1. Most common congenital abnormality of small intestine

    2. Failure of vitelline duct obliteration in utero

B. Clinical features

    1. "True" diverticulum: contains all layers of GI tract

        a. On antimesenteric border

            i. Tip may be free-floating (75%) or attached to umbilicus (24%)

        b. Ectopic mucosa

            i. Pancreatic, gastric, duodenal, biliary

    2. Male predominance

    3. Rule of 2's

 Remember the rule of 2's in Meckel diverticulum.

        a. 2% of population

        b. 2% become symptomatic

        c. Presents within first 2 years of life

        d. 2 types of mucosa (ileal and ectopic)

        e. 2 feet from ileocecal valve

        f. 2 cm in size

C. Presentation

    1. Incidentally discovered

    2. Symptomatic

        a. Pediatric

            i. Bleeding (most common cause of GI bleeding in children)

               (1) Ulcer on bowel mucosa across from MD due to acid

               (2) Secretion from ectopic gastric mucosa in MD

            ii. Intussusception

            iii. Obstruction

        b. Adult

            i. Obstruction

            ii. Perforation

            iii. Pain (mimics acute appendicitis)

D. Diagnosis
   1. Bleeding scan during acute episodes
   2. Technetium-99 pertechnate scan
      a. Identifies ectopic gastric mucosa within MD
   3. CT
      a. Inflamed mass/abscess
E. Treatment
   1. Asymptomatic
      a. Adult: no further therapy
      b. Pediatric: resect, with/without appendectomy
   2. Symptomatic
      a. Amenable to laparoscopy
      b. Diverticulectomy alone if feasible
         i. May narrow lumen
      c. Limited SB resection with anastomosis
         i. Includes ulcer on SB side
         ii. Must be done for bleeding MD

V. Crohn Disease

A. Pathophysiology
   1. Chronic, immune, mediated inflammatory bowel disease
   2. Differs from ulcerative colitis (Table 17.1)
   3. Affects entire GI tract

TABLE 17.1	Comparison of Crohn Disease and Ulcerative Colitis	
Parameter	**Crohn Disease**	**Ulcerative colitis**
Etiology	Unknown	Unknown
Pathology	Transmural	Mucosal
Disease pattern	SB and/or colon	Colon
Therapy	Corticosteroids	Corticosteroids and/or sulfasalazine
Presentation	Abdominal pain	Rectal bleeding
Cancer risk	Low	High
Systemic (non-GI) manifestations	Unusual	Common

      a. Most common in small intestine and anus
- i. Small intestine involvement, usually distal ileum (80%)
- ii. Exclusive ileum (20%–30%)
- iii. Ileocecal (40%–50%)
- iv. Exclusive colon (20%)
- v. Rectal sparing (50%)
- vi. Anus involvement (30%)
- vii. Mouth, gastroduodenal, esophagus, and proximal small intestine (rare)

      b. Discontinuous (skip lesion)

      c. Transmural
- i. Leads to fibrosis, thickened wall, structure
- ii. Fistula
- iii. Perforation
- iv. Fat wrapping (mesenteric fat around bowel)
- v. Noncaseating granuloma

B. Etiology
1. Unknown
2. Proposed potential causes
   - **a.** Genetic (*NOD2* gene: 40 × risk, chromosome 16q)
   - **b.** Infectious (mycobacteria)
   - **c.** Autoimmune
   - **d.** Environmental

C. Epidemiology
1. Incidence
   - **a.** Risen progressively (constant in ulcerative colitis [UC])
   - **b.** Northern Europe and North America: 4–6/100,000
   - **c.** Higher among Jews
2. Age of onset
   - **a.** Bimodal distribution
     - i. 15–40 years old
     - ii. 50–80 years old
3. Family history
   - **a.** 67% concordance with monozygotic twin
   - **b.** 15 × risk for a first-degree relative
4. Risk factors
   - **a.** Smoking (2 × risk)
5. Gender: affects male and female equally

D. Clinical features
    1. Ileitis
    2. Ileocolitis
    3. Colitis
    4. Perianal disease
        a. Anal fissures and ulcerations
        b. Perianal fistula
        c. Anorectal abscess
        d. Anal stenosis, rectal stricture
        e. Hemorrhoid
    5. Gastroduodenal disease
        a. Granuloma gastritis
        b. Aphthous ulcers
    6. Oral lesions (common in children)
        a. Aphthous ulcers
        b. Mucogingivitis
        c. Mucosal tags
        d. Lip swelling
        e. Cheilitis
        f. Granulomatous sialadenitis
    7. Extraintestinal
        a. Skin
            i. Erythema nodosum
            ii. Erythema multiforme
            iii. Pyoderma gangrenosum
        b. Eyes
            i. Iritis
            ii. Uveitis
            iii. Conjunctivitis
        c. Joints
            i. Arthritis (migratory)
            ii. Ankylosing spondylitis
        d. Liver
            i. Primary sclerosing cholangitis (more common in UC)
        e. Pancreas
            i. Pancreatitis
        f. Blood
            i. Anemia
            ii. Thrombocytosis

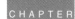

        iii. Arterial thrombosis

    g. General

        i. Amyloidosis

E. History and physical examination

    1. Diarrhea

    2. Abdominal pain

    3. Weight loss

    4. Growth failure in children

    5. Anorexia

    6. Fatigue

    7. Family history

    8. Recurrent perianal disease

    9. Right lower quadrant abdominal pain (mimics appendicitis)

F. Diagnosis

    1. Clinical suspicion

    2. Exclusion of differential diagnosis

        a. Peptic ulcer disease

        b. Lymphoma

        c. Appendicitis

        d. Infectious enteritis/colitis

        e. Diverticulitis

        f. Ischemic colitis

        g. Vasculitis

        h. Gynecologic disease

    3. Differentiate from UC

    4. Localization of disease

    5. Identification of extraintestinal manifestation

G. Laboratory tests

    1. Microcytic anemia

    2. Hypoalbuminemia

    3. Thrombocytosis

    4. Increase C-reactive protein

    5. Increase sedimentation rate

    6. ASCA positive: IgA and IgG to *Saccharomyces cerevisiae* (pANCA in UC)

H. Endoscopy

    1. Colonoscopy with ileoscopy

    2. Esophagogastroduodenoscopy (EGD)

    3. Capsule endoscopy

4. Push enteroscopy
I. Endoscopy findings
    1. Aphthous ulcers: deep/fissure ulcers, linear ulcers
    2. Cobblestoning ("cracks": deep linear ulcers, "stones": inflamed or normal tissue)
    3. Discontinuous lesions
    4. Nodular mucosa change
    5. Pseudopolyps (more common in UC)
    6. Normal rectum
    7. Normal vasculature adjacent to affected tissue
    8. Isolated involvement of terminal ileum (backwash ileitis with pancolitis in UC)
    9. Granuloma identified on biopsy
J. Imaging
    1. Barium study (barium swallow and SB follow-through)
        a. Cobblestone (linear ulcers, transverse sinuses and cleft)
        b. Segmental and irregular bowel involvement
        c. Ileal and cecal narrowing
        d. Fistula
    2. CT scan
        a. Transmural thickening
        b. Abscess
        c. Fistula
K. Treatment
    1. Treatment for acute exacerbation
        a. Bowel rest
        b. Parenteral nutrition
        c. Nasogastric suction for partial obstruction
        d. Antibiotic
        e. IV fluid
        f. Systemic steroid
        g. Surgery if medical treatment fails or acute complications develop
    2. Medical treatment
        a. Symptom control
            i. Antidiarrheal agents
        b. Corticosteroid (induction)
            i. Prednisone: steroid-dependent maintenance
            ii. Budesonide: only effective in ileum and cecum; less toxic

c. Aminosalicylates (maintenance)
  i. Sulfasalazine: colon disease
  ii. Mesalamine: SB disease and ileocolitis
  iii. Enema
d. 6-mercaptopurine (6-MP) and azathioprine
  i. Refractory patient (60%–70% response rate)
  ii. Fistula disease
e. Infliximab (chimeric mouse/human monoclonal antibody to tumor necrosis factors [TNF]-α)
  i. Steroid-refractory patient
  ii. Fistula disease
f. Methotrexate
g. Others
  i. Cyclosporine
  ii. Tacrolimus
  iii. Injection of fibrin glue for fistula
3. Surgery
  a. Focus on symptomatic areas; avoid extensive resection
  b. Indications
    i. Failure of medical management
    ii. Complications
      (1) Obstruction (most common)
      (2) Perforation
      (3) Stricture
      (4) Fistula
      (5) Growth failure (children)
      (6) Bleeding (rare; usually colon)
    iii. Development of dysplasia or carcinoma
  c. Surgical options
    i. Stricturoplasty
    ii. Segmental resection with primary anastomosis
    iii. Total colectomy with ileorectal anastomosis
    iv. Total proctocolectomy with ileoanal anastomosis
    v. Subtotal colectomy with ileostomy (emergency situation)
    vi. Abdominoperineal resection with permanent end colostomy (severe anorectal disease)
4. Nutrition support
5. Psychiatric support
6. Colorectal cancer screening

L. Prognosis
   1. 50% of patients require surgery
   2. Postoperative recurrence: 70%–80% (asymptomatic)
   3. Reoperation in 5 years: 25%–30%
   4. Increase risk of colon cancer

MENTOR TIPS DIGEST

- "Do not let sun set on a complete SB obstruction." In cases of complete obstruction, resuscitate the patient, and then go to the operating room.
- Remember the rule of twos in Meckel diverticulum.

Resources

Egan LJ, Sandborn WJ. Advances in the treatment of Crohn's disease. Gastroenterology 126:1574–1581, 2004.

Ephgrave K. Extra-intestinal manifestations of Crohn's disease. Surgical Clinics of North America 87:673–80, 2007.

Hatzaras IJ. Palesty JA, Abir F, et al. Small-bowel tumors. Epidemiologic and clinical characteristics of 1260 cases from the Connecticut tumor registry. Archives of Surgery 142:229–235, 2007.

Schwartz SI. Principles of surgery. McGraw-Hill, 2004.

Chapter Self-Test Questions

Circle correct answer. After you have responded to questions, check your answers in Appendix A.

1. List guidelines that make up the Rule of 2's in Meckel diverticulum:

_____

_____

_____

_____

_____

_____

2. List three to four predisposing factors for SB lymphoma:

_____

_____

_____

_____

3. It is possible for skin to show signs in Crohn disease. What are some relevant lesions?

_____

_____

_____

See the testbank CD for more self-test questions.

18 CHAPTER

COLON

Yuri W. Novitsky, MD, and Lou Reines, MD

I. Anatomy
  A. Topography
    1. Extends (150 cm) from cecum to rectum
    2. Right colon
      a. Cecum (first 6 cm from ileocecal valve)
      b. Ascending colon
      c. Hepatic flexure
    3. Transverse colon
    4. Left colon
      a. Splenic flexure
      b. Descending colon
      c. Sigmoid colon
  B. Peritoneal attachments
    1. Cecum (intraperitoneal)
      a. Mostly attached to retroperitoneum
      b. Completely mobile in 25%
    2. Ascending colon and hepatic flexure
      a. Fused to posterior body wall
      b. Covered by peritoneum anteriorly, laterally, and medially
    3. Transverse colon
      a. Intraperitoneal
      b. Mobile
      c. Broad mesocolon fused with inferior wall of lesser sac
      d. Gastrocolic ligament connects to greater curve of stomach
    4. Splenic flexure
      a. Renocolic ligament

5. Descending colon
  a. Covered by peritoneum anteriorly
  b. Attached to posterolateral body wall
    i. White line of Toldt
6. Sigmoid colon
  a. Iliac part (fixed)
  b. Pelvic (mobile)
    i. Broad mesentery with left ureter passing at base
C. Colon wall
  1. Serosa
    a. Contains epiploic appendages (not present in small bowel or rectum)
  2. Muscularis propria
    a. Inner circular
    b. Outer longitudinal
      i. Three distinct bands: teniae coli (not present in small bowel or rectum)
  3. Submucosa
  4. Mucosa
    a. No villi (unlike small bowel)
D. Blood supply
  1. Superior mesenteric artery
    a. Ileocolic and right colic arteries
      i. To cecum and ascending colon
    b. Middle colic artery
      i. Proximal transverse colon
  2. Inferior mesenteric artery
    a. Left colic
      i. Distal transverse colon and splenic flexure
    b. Sigmoid artery (may be multiple)
      i. Sigmoid colon
    c. Superior rectal (hemorrhoidal) artery
      i. Distal sigmoid colon
  3. Marginal artery of Drummond
    a. Begins at ileocolic and terminates in superior rectal arteries
    b. Parallels mesenteric border (2–6 cm away)
    c. Series of arcades: vasa recta
      i. Short branches to medial/mesenteric side
      ii. Long branches to lateral/antimesenteric side

E. Venous drainage
   1. Parallels blood supply
   2. Superior mesenteric vein
      a. Drains blood from right and transverse colon
   3. Superior rectal vein
      a. Drains blood from descending and sigmoid colon
      b. Forms inferior mesenteric vein
F. Lymphatic drainage
   1. Lymph node groups
      a. Epicolic: subserosal, within intestinal wall
      b. Paracolic: along marginal artery
      c. Intermediate: along large (named) arteries
      d. Principal: along root of mesentery

II. Diverticular Disease of Colon

A. Epidemiology
   1. Most common acquired pathology of colon
   2. Increased prevalence in Western world
      a. Prevalence of 0.2% in Africa/Asia
   3. Increased frequency with age
      a. <10% in <40 year old
      b. >70% in 80 year old
B. Anatomic distribution
   1. Western world: left-sided (sigmoid)
   2. Africa/Asia: right-sided
C. Pathophysiology
   1. False diverticula (most common in right- and left-sided disease)
      a. Not all layers are present in diverticulum
      b. Pulsion type
   2. Protrudes through areas of vasa recta penetration
   3. Associated with elevated intraluminal pressure
      a. Low-dietary fiber
      b. Hard stools (chronic constipation)
D. Disease spectrum
   1. Asymptomatic diverticular disease
      a. Diverticulosis (may be a cause of lower GI bleed, especially on right side)
   2. Symptomatic diverticular disease
      a. Acute diverticulitis

    i. Uncomplicated
      (1) Inflammation of colon wall and surrounding tissue
    ii. Complicated
      (1) Microperforation (abscess): common (approx 90% cases)
      (2) Macroperforation: (free air and peritonitis): uncommon (approx 10% cases)
      (3) Feculent peritonitis
      (4) Obstruction
      (5) Fistula

E. Natural history

  1. First attack

    a. 10%–25% lifetime risk of diverticulitis in patients with diverticulosis

    b. 15%–25% have complicated diverticulitis at first presentation

  2. Second attack

    a. 20%–30% will have recurrent diverticulitis

    b. 40%–60% will have complications

  3. Third attack

    a. Likely to recur again

F. Clinical presentation

 Sigmoid diverticulitis presents as "left-sided appendicitis," with left lower quadrant pain, fever, and leukocytosis.

  1. History

    a. Abdominal pain (85%)

    b. Diarrhea (80%)

    c. Nausea (18%)

    d. Bloody stools (15%)

    e. Constipation (5%–9%)

  2. Physical examination

    a. Fever

    b. Left lower quadrant tenderness

      i. May be suprapubic or right lower quadrant, given sigmoid colon mobility

    c. Palpable mass (some cases)

        d. Local peritoneal signs

        e. Diffuse peritoneal signs in severe complicated disease

    3. Laboratory findings

        a. Leukocytosis (11,000–25,000 range)

G. Differential diagnosis

    1. Inflammatory bowel disease

    2. Ischemic colitis

    3. Colon cancer (CA)

    4. Renal colic

    5. Gynecologic disorders

    6. Irritable bowel disease (in mild cases)

H. Imaging

    1. Computed tomography

        a. Intravenous and oral contrast

        b. Findings

            i. Diverticula

            ii. Inflamed colon

            iii. Thickened wall, pericolonic fat streaking (dirty fat)

            iv. Inflammatory mass, microperforation, pericolonic abscess

            v. Free air

I. Management

    1. Asymptomatic diverticulosis

        a. No treatment needed

        b. High-fiber diet

        c. No definitive evidence to avoid seeds, nuts, berries

    2. Acute diverticulitis: approximately 80% of cases respond to medical management

        a. Mild attack

            i. Oral antibiotics as outpatient

            ii. Clear liquids until symptoms improve

    3. Moderate/severe attack

        a. Intravenous hydration

        b. Bowel rest (nothing by mouth)

        c. Intravenous broad-spectrum antibiotics

            i. Cover gram-negative rods and anaerobes

        d. Percutaneous drainage of abscess (>5 cm)

J. Indications for surgery

    1. Elective

    a. Two to three documented episodes of uncomplicated diverticulitis

    b. One episode of complicated diverticulitis

  2. Emergent

    a. Free perforation with diffuse peritonitis

    b. Failure of conservative management/clinical deterioration

    c. Obstruction

    d. Abscess not amenable to percutaneous drainage

K. Surgical options

  1. Three-stage approach: rarely indicated in modern surgery

    a. Diverting colostomy

    b. Sigmoid resection

    c. Restoration of colonic continuity

  2. Two-stage approach: for acute complicated episode

    a. Sigmoid resection with colostomy and Hartmann pouch

    b. Restoration of colonic continuity

  3. Sigmoid resection with primary anastomosis (for elective cases)

    a. Amenable to laparoscopy in experienced hands

L. Perioperative considerations

  1. Inflammatory mass during emergent resections must be presumed malignant

  2. Mandatory colonoscopy (or contrast study) prior to elective resection

  3. Consider ureteral stenting to facilitate intraoperative ureter identification

  4. Mobilize splenic flexure to provide for tension-free anastomosis

  5. No indications for pelvic drainage postoperatively in elective setting

  6. Sigmoid resection margins

    a. Proximal: healthy colon

      i. No need to resect all diverticular

      ii. Avoid diverticula in anastomosis

    b. Distal: rectum

      i. Colorectal anastomosis to avoid recurrent diverticulitis

  7. Contraindications to primary anastomosis during emergent resections

    a. Patient instability

     b. Diffuse feculent spillage

     c. Diseased/inflamed intestinal segments at resection margin

     d. Frail state, immunosuppression, steroids

III. Large-Bowel Obstruction

  A. Etiology

     1. Mechanical obstruction

       a. Mass effect (leading three causes: colon CA, diverticulitis, volvulus)

     2. Adynamic (pseudo-) obstruction

       a. Autonomic dysfunction

         i. Risk factors: trauma, surgery (orthopedic, gynecologic, transplant), infection (pulmonary, urinary), metabolic (electrolyte abnormalities, uremia), pharmacologic (narcotics, antidepressants, anticholinergics), neuro-muscular disorders, pregnancy

  B. Pathophysiology

     1. Mechanical obstruction of colonic lumen

     2. Distention of proximal bowel

       a. Swallowed air

       b. Gas produced by gut bacteria

       c. Stool and gastrointestinal (GI) secretions

     3. Increase in colonic wall tension

       a. Highest in cecum due to largest diameter (Laplace law)

     4. Decreased mesenteric venous outflow in torsed mesentery

     5. Arterial insufficiency

       a. Mucosal ulcerations

       b. Transmural necrosis

       c. Perforation

  C. Clinical presentation

     1. Distention, vague central abdominal pain (not as dramatic as small-bowel obstruction)

     2. Investigate underlying illness, medication use, recent surgery/trauma, recent changes in bowel habits, previous episodes, constitutional problems

  D. History

     1. Obstipation

     2. Constipation

     3. Abdominal pain

  4. Emesis (late sign)

  5. Weight loss

  6. Blood in stool, melena

E. Physical examination

  1. Fever, tachycardia

  2. Abdominal examination

   a. Distention

   b. Tenderness (peritoneal signs usually not present)

   c. Ventral/groin hernia

  3. Rectal examination

   a. Mass

   b. Empty rectal vault

   c. Fecal impaction

F. Imaging

  1. Abdominal plain films

   a. Distended large bowel (haustrations)

   b. Collapsed distal bowel

   c. Paucity of rectal air

   d. Constipation

   e. Relatively collapsed small bowel (competent ileocecal valve)

   f. Air/fluid levels in small bowel (incompetent ileocecal valve)

  2. Gastrograffin enema

   a. Test of choice for suspected large-bowel obstruction

   b. Defines level, type, and extent of obstruction

    i. True versus pseudo-obstruction

    ii. "Apple core": colon CA

    iii. "Birds beak": volvulus

   c. Contraindicated in peritonitis or suspected perforation

  3. Computed tomography

   a. Triple (oral/intravenous/rectal) contrast

   b. Abdominal mass

   c. Abdominal wall/groin hernia

   d. Distended/collapsed large bowel (transition zone)

   e. Fecal impaction

   f. Foreign body

   g. Bowel ischemia/necrosis

    i. Free fluid, free air, pneumatosis intestinalis

    h. Metastatic CA

       i. Liver mass(es)

       ii. Peritoneal studding

       iii. Ascites

G. Differential diagnosis

   1. Dynamic

     a. Colon CA (70%)

     b. Diverticular disease (15%)

     c. Volvulus (10%)

     d. Hernia (2%)

     e. Stricture (1%–2%)

     f. Foreign body ($<1\%$)

   2. Adynamic

     a. Pseudo-obstruction (Ogilvie syndrome)

     b. Colonic inertia

H. Treatment

   1. Initial resuscitation

     a. Aggressive hydration

     b. Bowel rest

     c. Intravenous antibiotics (if signs of systemic infection or preoperative)

     d. Considerations for nonoperative (endoscopic, pharmacologic) decompression

   2. Surgical options

     a. Obstructing colon CA

       i. Right

         (1) Right hemicolectomy with primary anastomosis

       ii. Left

         (1) Segmental resection with colostomy and Hartmann pouch

         (2) Segmental resection, intraoperative lavage, primary anastomosis

         (3) Subtotal colectomy

         (4) Colonic stenting, laser tumor ablation, tube decompression, colonic preparation with subsequent resection/anastomosis

         (5) Diverting colostomy/ileostomy (advanced/metastatic disease)

b. Volvulus
  i. Sigmoid (Fig. 18.1)
    (1) Endoscopic decompression: recurrence up to 90% without surgery
    (2) Emergent resection with colostomy and Hartmann pouch if evidence of bowel compromise
    (3) Endoscopic decompression, bowel preparation, followed by colonic resection with anastomosis
    (4) Colonic pexis (higher recurrence rate)

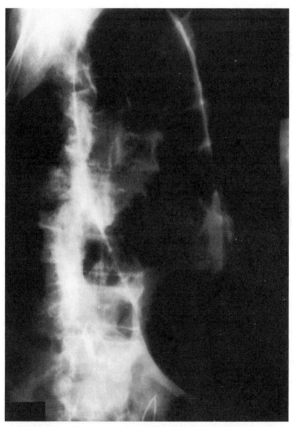

FIGURE 18.1 This plain film shows typical distended sigmoid colon filling most of abdomen in a sigmoid volvulus.

ii. Cecal
(1) Resection with ileostomy and mucous fistula
(2) Right hemicolectomy with anastomosis
(3) Cecopexy (30%–40% recurrence)

IV. Pseudo-obstruction (Ogilvie Syndrome)

A. Diagnosis of exclusion
  1. Must rule out mechanical obstruction
B. Treatment
  1. Initial management
   a. Bowel rest
   b. Intravenous fluids
   c. Rectal tube
   d. Gentle enemas
   e. Treatment of underlying cause
     i. Correction of electrolytes
     ii. Discontinue narcotics
  2. Endoscopic
   a. Decompression colonoscopy (with long tube placement)
  3. Pharmacologic
   a. Neostigmine (parasympathetic agonist)
     i. Effective in 70%–95%
     ii. Administer in a monitored setting (observe for brady-cardia)
   b. Guanethidine (adrenergic blocker)
   c. Naloxone (opiate antagonist)
  4. Surgery
   a. Reserved for medical failures or clinical deterioration
   b. Cecostomy (under local anesthesia)
   c. Blowhole loop cecostomy
   d. Segmental resection with ileostomy/mucous fistula if bowel compromised

V. Ulcerative Colitis (UC)

A. Pathophysiology
  1. Chronic, diffuse inflammatory disease
  2. Affects colon and rectum
   a. Continuous disease (begins distally)
     i. Rectum involvement (100%)

> The rectum is always involved (never spared) in cases of UC.

  ii. Anus spared (involved in Crohn disease)
 b. Confined to mucosa/submucosa
  i. Superficial ulcers
  ii. Friable mucosa with increased vascularity
   (1) No submucosal inflammation, thickening, fibrosis (Crohn)
  iii. Pseudopolyps
  iv. Crypt abscesses
  v. No transmural involvement
   (1) May occur in toxic megacolon

B. Etiology
 1. Remains unclear
 2. Proposed predisposing factors
  a. Bacterial/viral infection
  b. Autoimmune disease
  c. Genetic influence
  d. Environmental influence

C. Epidemiology
 1. Incidence
  a. Northern Europe, United States: 8–12/100,000
  b. Australia/South Africa: 4–6/100,000
  c. Asia/South America: <1/100,000
  d. Whites: 4 times non-whites
  e. Jews: 2–4 times non-Jews
 2. Age of onset
  a. Bimodal distribution (most 18–30 years old; second peak 45–55 years old)
  b. >60 years: rare (3%–5%)
 3. Family history
  a. 10%–25% with first-degree relatives

D. Clinical features
 1. Colitis
  a. Segmental, no skip areas (distal): 80%
  b. Pancolitis (20%)

    2. Extracolonic manifestations (15%–20%)
      a. Ocular involvement (parallels colitis)
      b. Uveitis, iritis, conjunctivitis, retinitis
      c. Articular (parallels colitis)
        i. Ankylosing spondylitis
        ii. Migratory arthritis (lower extremities)
        iii. Sacroiliitis
    3. Skin and oral cavity
      a. Pyoderma granulosum
      b. Aphthous stomatitis/erythema nodosum (rare)
    4. Liver and biliary tract (persists/progresses despite colectomy)
      a. Pericholangitis (80%)
      b. Sclerosing cholangitis (1%–4%)
      c. Progressive liver failure
E. History
    1. Bloody diarrhea
    2. Abdominal pain
    3. Weight loss
    4. Anorexia
    5. Extracolonic symptoms
F. Physical examination
    1. Fever, tachycardia
    2. Abdominal distention
    3. Abdominal tenderness (localized or diffuse)
    4. Anal sparing
    5. Must look for extracolonic manifestations
G. Differential diagnosis
    1. Diagnosis of exclusion
    2. Crohn disease (may be difficult to distinguish)
    3. Infectious colitis
      a. *Salmonella*
      b. *Shigella*
      c. *Campylobacter*
      d. *Escherichia coli*
      e. *Clostridium difficile*
      f. Parasites
      g. Viral
    4. Acute diverticulitis
    5. Ischemic colitis
    6. Colon CA

H. Imaging: no pathognomonic features for UC
   1. Barium enema (avoid if toxic megacolon is suspected)
      a. Mucosal granularity
      b. Burned-out colon (advanced chronic disease)
         i. Shortening of colon
         ii. Narrow caliber
         iii. Loss of redundancy
         iv. Disappearance of haustrations
         v. Mucosal atrophy
         vi. Pseudopolyps
         vii. Colonic dilation
            (1) "Toxic megacolon": transverse colon (80%–90%)
I. Endoscopy
   1. Loss of normal vascularity
   2. Friable mucosa with petechiae
   3. Ulcerations with surrounding raised granulation tissue (pseudopolyps)
   4. Must biopsy to differentiate from Crohn disease, ischemic colitis, or infectious colitis
J. Treatment
   1. Medical treatment for acute exacerbation
      a. Bowel rest
      b. Intravenous fluids
      c. Parenteral nutrition
      d. Systemic steroids
   2. Medical treatment for chronic disease
      a. Symptom control
         i. Antidiarrheal
         ii. Antispasmodic
      b. Anti-inflammatory
         i. 5-ASA compounds (oral or enemas)
         ii. Steroids
      c. Immunomodulators
         i. Azathioprine
         ii. Remicade
         iii. 6-Mercaptopurine
         iv. Methotrexate
         v. Cyclosporine
      d. Antibiotics
         i. Metronidazole

3. Indications for surgery
  a. Urgent/emergent
   i. Fulminant disease refractory to medical therapy (15%)
   ii. Toxic megacolon (5%–13%)
   iii. Free perforation (4%–10%)
   iv. Major hemorrhage (1%)
  b. Elective
   i. Failure of medical management (most common)
   ii. Development of dysplasia or frank carcinoma (2%–30%)
   iii. Stricture (11%)
   iv. Growth retardation (children)
4. Surgical options (Table 18.1)
  a. Emergent
   i. Subtotal colectomy with ileostomy
   ii. Proctocolectomy with ileostomy
  b. Elective
   i. Proctocolectomy with end ileostomy
   ii. Proctocolectomy with Kock (continent) ileostomy

TABLE 18.1

Advantages and Disadvantages of Reconstruction Options for Ulcerative Colitis

Procedure	Advantages	Disadvantages
Standard Brooke ileostomy*	Surgically simple, few complications	Patient wears permanent bag.
Continent ileostomy*	No constant fecal leakage	Patient must periodically intubate and drain.
Ileoanal pull-through†	Maintains anal sphincter, no "ostomy"	Patients have 4–10 bowel movements daily; sometimes there is nocturnal leakage.

*Older patients (>50 years) may wish to avoid reliving "potty training" and choose an ileostomy.

† In general, younger patients (<50 years) requiring total colectomy for ulcerative colitis should be offered an ileoanal pull-through.

      iii. Proctocolectomy with ileal pouch-anal anastomosis (procedure of choice)
5. Prognosis
    a. Long-term failure of medical management: 20%–30%
    b. Complications (see above)
    c. CA risk

> Patients with active ulcerative colitis (UC) for 10 years have a 2-3% incidence of colon CA. This percentage rises 1%–2% per year thereafter.

      i. 2%–3% first 10 years
      ii. 1%–2% per year afterwards
    d. Operative mortality
      i. Elective (1%–3%)
      ii. Emergent: 10%

VI. Colon CA
  A. Epidemiology
    1. Fourth most common malignancy
    2. Adenocarcinoma (most common type)
    3. 150,000 new cases annually in United States
    4. 57,000 annual deaths
    5. More common in industrialized countries
  B. Pathogenesis/risk factors
    1. Dietary (high animal fat, low fiber)
    2. Mutagenesis (*ras* proto-oncogene, *APC, p53*)
    3. Inflammatory bowel disease
    4. Familial
    5. Adenomatous polyposis (FAP), Gardner syndrome
    6. Nonpolyposis (Lynch syndrome)
  C. Colonic polyps
    1. Non-neoplastic: no malignant potential
      a. Hyperplastic, inflammatory, juvenile, hamartomatous
    2. Neoplastic: may progress to dysplasia and carcinoma
      a. CA risk increases with size
        i. Tubulous polyp (75%)
          (1) 5% chance of malignancy
        ii. Tubulovillous polyp (15%)
          (1) 22% chance of malignancy

        iii. Villous polyp (10%)

           (1) 40% chance of malignancy

D. Prevention/screening

  1. General population

    a. Annual fecal occult blood test (FOBT)

      i. Positive results in 2%–10%

    b. Flexible sigmoidoscopy/barium enema (BE) every 5–10 years, or

    c. First screening colonoscopy at age of 50, then every 10 years

      i. 5% rate of missed polyps during screening

    d. Colonoscopy for positive FOBT, sigmoidoscopy, or BE

    e. After polypectomy, repeat colonoscopy after 3 years or sooner

  2. High-risk population

    a. First-degree relative with known hereditary colon CA: colonoscopy at age 20 years

    b. Ulcerative colitis: colonoscopy 10 years after disease onset

    c. Family history of colon CA: colonoscopy at age of 40 years

E. Presentation

  1. Asymptomatic (incidentally discovered)

  2. Symptomatic

    a. Intermittent pain

    b. Bleeding

    c. Melena (right-sided lesions)

    d. Change in bowel habits

    e. Constipation

    f. Decreased stool caliber

    g. Obstructions (more commonly left-sided)

    h. Perforation

F. Diagnosis

  1. Digital rectal examination

    a. Palpation of distal masses

    b. Stool sampling for blood

  2. Flexible sigmoidoscopy

    a. For rectum and sigmoid

  3. Barium contrast enema

    a. 85%–92% sensitive to detect polyps

4. Computed tomography
    a. Oral contrast needed
    b. More useful for detection of metastatic disease
5. Colonoscopy
    a. Only means of tissue diagnosis
    b. 0.1%–0.3% rate of perforation/hemorrhage
G. Treatment
    1. Polyp
        a. Endoscopic resection
        b. Surgical resection if not amenable to endoscopic means
            i. Local resection via colotomy (for small benign polyps only)
            ii. Regional resection (with frozen section exclusive of malignancy)
            iii. Formal segmental resection (see following)
    2. Malignant polyp
        a. Complete removal
        b. Cure if no penetration of muscularis mucosae (carcinoma in situ)
    3. Invasive CA
        a. Segmental resection
        b. Adjuvant (postoperative) chemotherapy for node-positive lesions
H. Staging
    1. Various classifications based on depth of invasion, lymph-node status, and distant metastasis
        a. Tumor node metastasis (TNM) system
        b. Duke classification (Table 18.2)

TABLE 18.2		
Duke Classification of Colorectal CA		
Class	**Depth**	**5-Year Survival Rate**
A	Limited to muscularis	90%
B1	Through muscularis	70%
B2	Through muscularis to serosa	50%
C	Any depth with positive nodes	30%–40%
D	Distal metastasis	<20%

I. Location-based surgical considerations
  1. Right-sided colon CA (15%)
    a. Right hemicolectomy
      i. Mesentery margin
        (1) Ileocolic artery
        (2) Right colic artery
        (3) Right branch of middle colic artery
      ii. Colon margin
        (1) 10 cm of distal terminal ileum
        (2) Mid-transverse colon
      iii. Anastomosis
        (1) Ileum to mid-transverse colon
  2. Transverse colon CA (8%)
    a. Extended right hemicolectomy/splenic flexure resection
      i. Mesentery margin
        (1) Ileocolic artery
        (2) Right colic artery
        (3) Middle colic artery
      ii. Colon margin
        (1) 10 cm of distal terminal ileum
        (2) Proximal descending colon
      iii. Anastomosis
        (1) Ileum to left or sigmoid colon
  3. Descending colon/splenic flexure CA (5%)
    a. Left hemicolectomy
      i. Mesentery margin
        (1) Left branch of middle colic artery
        (2) Left colic artery
      ii. Colon margin
        (1) Mid-transverse colon
        (2) Proximal sigmoid colon
      iii. Anastomosis
        (1) Mid-transverse to sigmoid colon
  4. Sigmoid colon CA (70%)
    a. Sigmoid resection (low-anterior resection)
      i. Mesentery margin
        (1) Left colic artery
        (2) Sigmoid arteries
        (3) Superior rectal artery

    ii. Colon margin

       (1) Distal descending colon

       (2) Upper rectum

    iii. Anastomosis

       (1) Descending colon to rectum

J. Laparoscopic colectomy for CA

    1. Proven modality for all locations

    2. Safe and effective if oncologic principles followed

    3. Improved perioperative outcomes

    4. No long-term differences in disease-related outcomes

    5. Possible survival advantage in laparoscopic patients with stage IIIA

K. Postoperative surveillance

    1. History/physical

      a. Every 3 months for 3 years, then annually

    2. Carcinoembryonic antigen (CEA) levels

      a. With history/physical, investigate if elevated

    3. Colonoscopy

      a. 1-year postoperatively

      b. If normal, every 3–5 years

    4. Not indicated

      a. Complete blood count

      b. Liver function test

      c. FOBT

      d. Chest radiography

      e. Computed tomography

L. Prognosis

    1. Overall 5-year survival: 62%

    2. Local recurrence following resection

      a. Stages I and II: 20%

      b. Stages III and IV: 50%–65%

        i. 50% within 18 months

        ii. 90% within 3 years

      c. Re-resection: 18%–30%; mean 5-year survival

    3. Distant metastasis (17% at initial presentation)

      a. Liver (most frequent site): 15%–24%

        i. Resection (if no extrahepatic tumor, fewer than four lesions in one lobe)

        ii. 5-year survival: 25%–30%

          iii. Unresectable: systemic/local chemotherapy

          iv. Poor prognosis

    b. Lung (10%)

        i. Usually in setting of liver metastasis

        ii. Resection: 20% 5-year survival

M. Clinically validated (adverse) prognostic indicators for colon CA

  1. Local extent of tumor

    a. Mesothelial inflammatory and/or hyperplastic reaction with tumor close to serosal surface

    b. Tumor present at serosal surface with an inflammatory reaction, mesothelial hyperplasia, and/or erosion or ulceration

    c. Free tumor cells on serosal surface within peritoneum, with underlying ulceration of visceral peritoneum

  2. Regional node involvement

    a. Both positive and negative nodes are important

    b. Total number of lymph nodes in surgical specimen directly influences accuracy of nodal staging and prognosis (relapse-free and overall 5-year survival)

    c. ≥14 nodes: 81% and 82%, respectively

    d. 9–13 nodes: 72%–74%, respectively

    e. 5–8 nodes: 66%–71%, respectively

    f. <5 nodes: 63%–68%, respectively

  3. Vascular invasion

  4. Residual tumor following definitive therapy

  5. Serum CEA

    a. Preoperative serum levels of tumor marker CEA that are 5.0 ng/mL or above have an adverse impact on survival that is independent of tumor stage.

  6. Tumor grade

    a. Histologic grade reflects extent of tumor differentiation

  7. Circumferential (radial) margins

MENTOR TIPS DIGEST

- Sigmoid diverticulitis presents as "left-sided appendicitis," with left lower quadrant pain, fever, and leukocytosis.
- The rectum is always involved (never spared) in cases of UC.
- Patients with active ulcerative colitis (UC) for 10 years have a 3% incidence of colon CA. This percentage rises 1%–2% per year thereafter.

Resources

Corman ML, ed. Colon and rectal surgery. Lipincott Williams and Wilkins, 2004.

Evans J, Kozol R, Lukianoff A, et al. Does a 48-hour rule predict outcomes in acute sigmoid diverticulitis? Journal of Gastrointestinal Surgery 12:577–582, 2008.

Kozol RA, Hyman N, Strong S, et al. Minimizing risk in colorectal surgery. American Journal of Surgery 194:576–587, 2007.

Chapter Self-Test Questions

Circle the correct answer. After you have responded to questions, check your answers in Appendix A.

1. Which segments of the colon lie in a retroperitoneal position?

   a. Ascending colon

   b. Sigmoid colon

   c. Descending colon

   d. Both A and C

2. How long is a completely developed colon in an adult?

   a. 3 m

   b. 1.5 m

   c. 2 m

   d. 0.5 m

3. What area of the colon is particularly susceptible to vascular insult as it is considered a watershed area?

   a. Splenic flexure

   b. Cecum

   c. Hepatic flexure

   d. Descending colon

4. What type of nutrient represents the main source of energy for the colon?

   a. Glutamine

   b. N-butyrate

   c. Leucine

   d. Sucrose

5. A large population of colonic bacteria comprises up to 90% of the dry weight of feces. Which type of bacteria dominate in the colon?

   a. Gram-positive cocci

   b. Gram-positive rods

   c. Gram-negative rods

   d. Anaerobes

See the testbank CD for more self-test questions.

19

ANORECTUM

Yuri W. Novitsky, MD, and Louis Reines, MD

I. Anatomy
   A. Rectum
      1. Length: about 12–14 cm
         a. Extends from sacral promontory to levator ani muscle
      2. Circumferential coverage by outer longitudinal muscles
      3. No taeniae coli
      4. Three lateral curves: submucosal folds (valves of Houston)
         a. Left inferior (10–12 cm from anal verge)
         b. Right middle (8–10 cm from anal verge)
         c. Left superior (4–7 cm from anal verge)
      5. Peritoneum and attachments
         a. Covers upper ⅔ anteriorly (6–8 cm from anal verge)
         b. Covers upper ⅓ laterally
         c. Posterior rectum: devoid of peritoneum
            i. Endopelvic fascia (attaches to sacrum)
            ii. Lateral rectal stalks
   B. Anal canal
      1. Length: about 3 cm
      2. Layers of wall
         a. Smooth muscle
            i. Inner: circular (forms internal sphincter)
            ii. Outer: longitudinal
         b. Wrapped by striated muscle (external sphincter)
         c. Arranged in three U-shaped loops
            i. Subcutaneous (surrounds anus, attached to perianal skin)
            ii. Superficial: anococcygeal ligament (attaches to coccyx)

      iii. Deep: puborectalis muscle (attaches to pubis)

      iv. Form efficient anal closure

  d. Mucosa

3. Perianal area: pigmented skin, sebaceous glands, hair follicles

  a. Squamous epithelium (below dentate line)

     i. Location of internal hemorrhoidal plexus

  b. Columnar epithelium (above dentate line)

  c. Transitional zone: up to 1 cm above dentate line

     i. Columnar, transitional, or squamous epithelium

4. Dentate (pectinate) line: about midpoint of canal

  a. Most important landmark

  b. 2 cm from anal verge

  c. Formed by margins of anal valves and longitudinal mucosal folds of Morgagni

  d. Transition between visceral (above) and somatic (below) areas

  e. Implications for arterial supply, venous lymphatic drainage, nerve supply, associated disease (squamous cell carcinoma versus adenocarcinoma

5. Perianorectal spaces

  a. Potential spaces filled with fat

  b. May be site of infection/abscess

6. Perianal space

  a. Surrounds anus

  b. Contiguous with subcutaneous fat of buttocks

7. Ischioanal space (paired)

  a. Triangular region between external sphincter (medially), levator ani muscle (superiorly), ischium (laterally), and ischiorectal fossa septum (inferiorly)

  b. Contains fat, inferior rectal vessels, and lymphatics

  c. Both sides may be connected by deep postanal space

  d. Site of a horseshoe abscess

8. Intersphincteric space

  a. Between external and internal sphincters

  b. Connects to perianal space inferiorly

  c. May be contiguous with rectal wall superiorly

9. Supralevator space

  a. Above levator ani muscle

  b. Boarded by peritoneal reflection superiorly

    c. Communicates posteriorly, may allow infectious spread into retroperitoneum

C. Arterial supply

    1. Superior rectal artery (from inferior mesenteric artery)

        a. Bifurcates at posterior rectum into left and right branches

        b. Supplies rectum and upper portion of anal canal (above dentate line)

    2. Middle rectal arteries (from internal iliac arteries)

        a. Supplies lower rectum

        b. Prostate gland

    3. Inferior rectal arteries (from internal pudendal arteries)

        a. Supplies distal anal canal and anal sphincter muscles

    4. Median sacral artery (from aorta)

        a. Few small branches to posterior rectum

D. Venous drainage

    1. Portal system (via inferior mesenteric vein)

        a. Superior rectal vein: rectum and upper anus

    2. Systemic system (via internal iliac veins)

        a. Middle rectal veins: lower part of rectum and upper anal canal

        b. Inferior rectal veins: lower anal canal

    3. Anastomosis between two systems forms portosystemic shunt

E. Lymphatic drainage

    1. Rectum

        a. Upper/middle

            i. To mesenteric nodes along superior rectal artery

        b. Lower

            i. To mesenteric nodes along superior rectal artery

            ii. To internal iliac nodes along middle rectal artery

    2. Anal canal

        a. Above dentate line

            i. To mesenteric nodes along superior rectal artery

            ii. To internal iliac nodes along middle rectal artery

        b. Below dentate line

            i. To internal iliac nodes along middle rectal artery

II. Rectal Cancer (CA)

A. Incidence

    1. 1%–2% lifetime risk

    2. 30% of colorectal CA

    3. 100,000 deaths annually

B. Risk factors
  1. Family history
  2. Ulcerative colitis
  3. Crohn disease
  4. Familial adenomatous polyposis (FAP)
C. Diagnosis
  1. History
    a. Blood per rectum
    b. Change in bowel habits/caliber
    c. Tenesmus
    d. Weight loss
    e. Abdominal pain
  2. Physical examination
    a. Palpable mass on rectal examination
  3. Imaging
    a. Computed tomography
      i. Depth of invasion
      ii. Nodal/distant metastasis
    b. Endorectal ultrasound: very sensitive/specific
      i. Depth of invasion
      ii. Nodal metastasis
D. Treatment
  1. Neoadjuvant therapy
    a. Tumor downstaging
    b. Decreased locoregional recurrence after surgery
    c. Possible survival benefit
  2. Adjuvant therapy
    a. Decreases local recurrence
    b. Improved survival
  3. Surgical therapy
    a. Local (transanal excision)
      i. Less than 6–8 cm from anal verge
      ii. Smaller than 4-cm lesions
      iii. Less than 1/3 of rectum in circumference
      iv. Mobile lesion
      v. No evidence of nodal disease
      vi. Poor surgical candidate
    b. Transanal endoscopic microsurgery (TEM)
      i. For tumors 8–12 cm from anal verge

   ii. CO_2-facilitated
   iii. Special equipment required
  c. Sphincter-preserving resections
   i. Total mesorectal excision (TME)
   ii. Coloanal anastomosis
   iii. Colonic J pouch
  d. Abdominoperineal resection (APR)
   i. For cancers close to anal verge
   ii. For patients with fecal incontinence
 E. Prognosis (5-year survival)
  1. Stage I: 72%
  2. Stage II: 52%
  3. Stage III: 37%
  4. Stage IV: 4%

III. Anal CA

 A. Epidemiology
  1. More common in females
  2. Sixth to seventh decades of life
 B. Etiology/risk factors
  1. Human papillomavirus (HPV) infection
  2. Anal-receptive intercourse
  3. Immunocompromised states
   a. HIV infection
   b. Transplant recipient
  4. Chronic anal fistula
  5. Crohn disease
 C. Presentation
  1. Varies by type
  2. Often late due to no or minimal symptoms
  3. High index of suspicion (30% misdiagnosed initially)
 D. History and physical examination
  1. Pruritus
  2. Pain
  3. Bleeding
  4. Indurated anal mass
 E. Diagnosis
  1. Digital rectal examination: most important
  2. Biopsy
  3. Endoscopic evaluation

      4. Endoluminal ultrasound

      5. Computed tomography

      6. Magnetic resonance imaging

   F. Differential diagnosis

      1. Crohn disease

      2. Hidradenitis suppurativa

      3. Idiopathic pruritus ani

      4. Condyloma acuminatum

   G. Clinical features of perianal neoplasms

      1. Squamous cell carcinoma (SCC)

         a. Similar to other skin SCC

         b. Indurations/ulcerations of perianal skin

         c. Often discovered at a later stage

         d. Size determines survival

      2. Basal cell carcinoma (BCC)

         a. Central ulceration with irregular, raised borders

      3. Bowen disease

         a. Intraepidermal SCC (in situ)

         b. Scaly or crusted plaque

         c. Progressed to SCC if untreated

      4. Perianal Paget disease

         a. Eczematous perianal skin rash with oozing or scaling

         b. Paget cells on biopsy

         c. Often metastatic at presentation

      5. Verrucous carcinoma

         a. Large, soft, painful, wart-like growth (cauliflower appearance)

         b. Aggressive local growth with erosion/pressure necrosis of surrounding tissues

   H. Treatment of perianal neoplasms

      1. Wide local excision

      2. Negative microscopic margins

      3. Re-excise local BCC recurrence

      4. Abdominoperineal resection (APR)

         a. Reserved for selected patients

         b. Large lesions

         c. Anal incontinence/sphincter involvement

         d. Uncontrollable local recurrence

      5. Chemoradiation for advanced SCC

IV. Anal Canal Neoplasms
A. SCC
1. Clinical features may be similar to those of perianal lesions
2. Long-standing history of perianal problems
3. Inguinal metastasis in 15%–45% of patients
   a. May be diagnosed by physical examination or sentinel node biopsy
4. Wide local excision for early (<2 cm) lesions only
   a. No role for prophylactic inguinal lymphadenectomy
5. Chemoradiation (Nigro protocol) for lesions >2 cm
   a. Including involved inguinal regions, if nodal disease present
6. APR (limited role)
   a. Chemoradiation failure
   b. Fecal incontinence
B. Adenocarcinoma
1. Rectal type
   a. Similar to colon CA
2. Anal glands
   a. From columnar epithelium of anal gland ducts
   b. Often extramucosal
3. Risk factors
   a. Anorectal fistula
   b. Long-standing perianal disease
4. Treatment
   a. Local resection of small superficial rectal-type lesions
      i. APR for all other lesions, with or without groin lymph node dissection
      ii. Chemoradiation (Nigro protocol) for select patients
C. Anal melanoma
1. Rare malignant neoplasm
2. Third commonest site of melanoma
3. Arises from epidermoid lining of anal canal
4. Rectal bleeding most common symptom
5. High likelihood of submucosal spread
6. Spreads to mesenteric lymph nodes
7. Hematogenous spread to liver and lungs (cause of death)
8. Treatment
   a. Local excision

       b. APR for select patients

       c. Prognosis extremely poor

  D. Prognosis

     1. Perianal neoplasms

       a. SCC

          i. 100% cure for superficial and small lesions

          ii. 60% 5-year survival for lesion larger than 2 cm

       b. BCC

          i. 70% 5-year survival

       c. Paget disease

          i. Poor prognosis due to late presentation

     2. Anal canal neoplasms

       a. SCC

          i. 70%–90% 5-year survival

       b. Melanoma

          i. Very poor

V. Hemorrhoids

  A. Downward displacement of anal cushions in submucosa underlying squamocolumnar transition zone of anal canal

  B. Constant anatomic location

     1. Left lateral, right anterior, right posterior

  C. Etiology

     1. Constipation

     2. Weakened/fragmented supporting tissue of anal cushions

     3. Explosive diarrhea

     4. Prolonged labor

  D. Classification

     1. External hemorrhoid (EH)

       a. Dilated venules of inferior hemorrhoidal plexus below dentate line

       b. Covered by squamous epithelium

       c. May form a clot in plexus: thrombosed EH

     2. Internal hemorrhoid (IH)

       a. Anal cushions above dentate line

       b. Covered by columnar epithelium

       c. Classification of IH

          i. First degree: anal cushions slide beyond dentate line

          ii. Second degree: prolapse through anus on straining; reduce spontaneously

    iii. Third degree: prolapse through anus on straining, reduced manually

    iv. Fourth degree: prolapse through anus; not reducible

E. Clinical presentation

 Internal hemorrhoids generally do not cause pain. The most common problem caused by internal hemorrhoids is rectal bleeding.

  1. History

    a. Painless rectal bleeding with defecation due to trauma to mucosa overlying hemorrhoid

    b. Itching

  2. Physical examination

    a. EH: congested tissue (very painful if thrombosed)

    b. IH: cannot be palpated

F. Diagnosis

  1. Visual inspection

  2. Digital rectal examination

    a. Examination under anesthesia (EUA) if too painful

  3. Anoscopy/proctoscopy

G. Differential diagnosis

  1. If pain present: pruritus ani, anal fissure, abscess are more likely

  2. Painless bleeding: colitis, arteriovenous malformation, CA

    a. Must rule out a proximal gastrointestinal (GI) source

H. Treatment

  1. Thrombosed EH

    a. Excision (preferable)

    b. Incision/evacuation of clot

  2. IH

    a. High-fiber diet (first, second degree)

    b. Sclerotherapy (no longer popular)

      i. 60%–80% effective

      ii. 30% recurrence rate at 4 years

    c. Rubber-band ligation (first, second, some third degree)

      i. One or two hemorrhoids per session

      ii. Minimal procedural discomfort

iii. Contraindicated in immunosuppressed
    (1) Post-procedure excessive pain, fever, urinary retention: rule out pelvic sepsis
iv. 70%–100% effective
v. Recurrence in up to 70%
vi. Amenable to repeat banding

d. Thermal control, infrared photocoagulation
    i. 70%–95% effective in controlling bleeding

e. Hemorrhoidectomy
    i. Indications
      (1) Severe prolapse
      (2) Recurrent thrombosis
      (3) Intractability (frequent bleeding)
      (4) Strangulation with/without ulceration
      (5) Hygienic difficulty
    ii. Techniques
      (1) Open hemorrhoidectomy (rare)
      (2) Closed hemorrhoidectomy (most common)
      (3) Stapled hemorrhoidopexy (procedure for prolapse and hemorrhoids) (PPH) (newest)
    iii. Complications
      (1) Urinary retention (2%–36%)
      (2) Bleeding (0%–6%)
      (3) Anal stenosis (0%–6%)
      (4) Fecal incontinence (2%–12%)
      (5) Infection ($<5\%$)

VI. Anal Fissure

A. Ulceration of lower anal canal

B. Classification
  1. Primary: no associated illnesses
  2. Secondary: associated with Crohn disease, leukemia, aplastic anemia, agranulocytosis, AIDS, *Chlamydia,* syphilis, tuberculosis

C. Pathophysiology
  1. Hard stool
  2. Explosive diarrhea
  3. Anal trauma
  4. Increased anal sphincter tone

D. History
1. Constipation or difficult bowel movement
2. Significant anal pain: posterior midline (increased with defecation)
   a. Burning, throbbing, sharp in acute episodes
3. Bleeding (staining of toilet tissue)

E. Physical examination
1. Triad
   a. Ulcer in posterior midline
      i. Secondary fissurae lateral
   b. Sentinel pile: fibrotic skin tag
   c. Hypertrophic anal papilla

F. Diagnosis
1. Visual inspection
2. Digital rectal examination (painful)
   a. EUA if too painful
3. Anoscopy/proctoscopy
4. Biopsy of fissure and rectal mucosa (for suspected secondary fissures)

G. Differential diagnosis
1. Anal fistula
2. Anal abrasion
3. Hemorrhoids
4. Anal cancer

H. Treatment
1. Acute fissure
   a. 70% heal spontaneously
   b. 30% become chronic
2. Initial therapy
   a. Pain relief
   b. Anal hygiene (warm sitz bath)
   c. Stool bulk-forming agents
3. Local therapy (to reduce anal resting pressure)
   a. Topical 0.4% nitroglycerin paste
   b. Botulinum toxin (Botox) injections
   c. Topical calcium-channel blockers (nifedipine)
4. Surgical therapy: 98% effective
   a. Internal sphincterotomy (gold standard)
   b. Open or closed technique

    c. Fissurectomy with anoplasty

    d. Avoid surgery for secondary fistulas

VII. Anorectal Abscess

  A. Prevalence

    1. Less than 5% lifetime risk

  B. Pathogenesis

    1. Infection of anal glands at dentate line (cryptoglandular)

    2. Infection spread to potential spaces (see preceding)

    3. Direct extension from intra-abdominal sources

      a. Crohn, diverticulitis, appendicular abscess

    4. Secondary superinfection in various settings

      a. Crohn disease

      b. Tuberculosis

      c. Lymphogranuloma venerum

      d. Trauma

      e. Foreign body

  C. Clinical features

    1. Location (decreasing frequency)

    2. Perianal, ischioanal, intersphincteric, supralevator

  D. Symptoms

    1. Anal pain

    2. Swollen mass

    3. Very painful rectal examination (perirectal abscess)

    4. Perianal drainage

    5. Fever

    6. Septicemia

  E. Diagnosis

    1. Visual inspection

    2. Digital rectal examination

      a. EUA if too painful

    4. Anoscopy/proctoscopy

  F. Treatment

    1. Important to differentiate between perianal and perirectal processes

    2. Perianal abscess

      a. Incision and drainage

      b. Curettage and irrigation of wound

      c. No packing needed, unless very extensive

      d. No antibiotics, unless immunocompromised or with cardiac/joint prosthetics

  3. Ischioanal (perirectal) abscess

      a. Originates in deep postanal space, spreads to both ischioanal spaces

      b. Drainage through deep postanal space

      c. Incise skin between coccyx and anus

      d. Incise anococcygeal ligament

      e. Curettage, irrigation, light packing for 24 hours

      f. Antibiotics if signs of systemic infection

  4. Intersphincteric abscess

      a. No external signs

      b. Severe pain; rectal examination impossible

      c. Transrectal incision and drainage

  5. Supralevator abscess

      a. Rare

      b. May mimic intra-abdominal process

      c. Treatment strategy according to site of origin

         i. From intersphincteric space: transrectal drainage

         ii. From ischiorectal space: drainage through ischioanal fossa

         iii. From intra-abdominal source: transrectal or trans-ischional drainage; treat underlying cause

G. Complications

  1. Sepsis (if untreated)

  2. Chronic fistula in 15%–40% of cases

VIII. Anal Fistula

A. Inflammatory track with internal opening in anal crypts and external opening in perianal skin

B. Pathogenesis

  1. Fistula often follows incompletely healed perianal abscess

  2. Trauma

  3. Foreign body

  4. Pelvic/intra-abdominal abscess

C. Classification

  1. Intersphincteric (70%)

      a. Begins at anal crypts, extends to intersphincteric plane

      b. Downward extension of track in intersphincteric plane

      c. External opening close to anal verge

    2. Transsphincteric (25%)

      a. Begins at anal crypts, extends to intersphincteric plane

      b. Lateral extension through external sphincter

      c. Downward extension toward external opening at ischioanal fossa

    3. Suprasphincteric (<5%)

      a. Begins at anal crypts, extends to intersphincteric plane

      b. Upward extension above puborectal muscle

      c. Downward extension through levator ani toward external opening at ischioanal fossa

    4. Extrasphincteric (<1%)

      a. Begins at rectal lumen

      b. Downward extension through levator ani toward external opening at ischioanal fossa

D. Clinical presentation

    1. Intermittent or persistent feculant drainage

    2. History of perianal abscess

    3. Recurrent perianorectal abscess

E. Diagnosis

    1. Visualization

      a. External opening with elevated granulation tissue

      b. Purulent or serosanguineous drainage may be expressed

    2. Digital rectal examination

      a. Fistulous track may be palpable as indurated cord

    3. Anoscopy

> Remember "posterior-midline" as a key idea in two respects: where 90% of anal fissures occurs, and a fistula-in-ano with an external opening that is posterior to a horizontal line bisecting anus has a curvilinear course with an internal opening at posterior midline.

      a. Identifies internal opening

    4. Proctoscopy/sigmoidoscopy

F. Differential diagnosis

    1. Hidradenitis suppurativa

    2. Pilonidal cyst/sinus

    3. Secondary fistula

    4. Crohn disease

    5. Ulcerative colitis

    6. Rectal carcinoma

    7. Anal carcinoma

G. Treatment

    1. Surgery (fistulotomy)

        a. Placing probe in fistula

        b. Opening fistulous track

        c. Curettage of granulation tissue of track

        d. Fistulotomy may cause anal incontinence

    2. Staged fistulotomy with Seton placement

    3. No need for fistulectomy

IX. Pilonidal Cyst

A. Infection of hair follicle in sacrococcygeal area

B. Located at 3–5 cm cephalad from anus

C. Cephalad extension of sinus

D. Epidemiology

    1. Hirsute male

    2. Overweight

    3. Second or third decade of life

E. Clinical manifestation

    1. Abscess (most common)

    2. Draining sinus

    3. Midline pits (infected hair follicle)

F. History

    1. Pain

G. Physical examination

    1. Tender fluctuant mass

    2. Surrounding cellulitis

    3. Sinus opening in chronic cases

H. Differential diagnosis

    1. Hidradenitis suppurativa

    2. Skin furuncle

    3. Anal fistula

    4. Syphilis

    5. Tuberculosis

    6. Actinomycosis

I. Treatment

  1. Acute

    a. Abscess incision (off midline) and drainage

    b. Light packing

  2. Chronic

    a. Excision of cyst with closure by secondary intention

      i. Recurrence up to 18%

      ii. Healing time 4–6 weeks

      iii. May result in chronically nonhealing wounds

    b. Excision of cyst with marsupialization

      i. Healing time 4 weeks

      ii. Recurrence 6%–15%

    c. Radical resection down to periosteum

      i. Recurrence rate 2%–13%

      ii. Healing time 8–21 weeks

      iii. Frequent nonhealing wounds

    d. Lateral approach

      i. Incision 2 cm off midline

      ii. Identification, incision, curettage of fistulous tracts/cavity

      iii. Open wound

        (1) Gauze or vacuum-based dressing

        (2) Rapid wound healing

        (3) Recurrence 7%–22%

    e. Flap procedures

      i. Technically difficult

      ii. Reserved for severe disease

 MENTOR TIPS DIGEST

- Internal hemorrhoids generally do not cause pain. The most common problem caused by internal hemorrhoids is rectal bleeding.
- Remember "posterior-midline" as key idea in two respects: where 90% of anal fissures occurs, and a fistula-in-ano with an external opening that is posterior to a horizontal line bisecting anus has a curvilinear course with an internal opening at posterior midline.

Resources

Corman ML, ed. Colon and Rectal Surgery. Lipincott Williams and Wilkins, 2004.

Kaidar-Person O. Hemorrhoidal disease: A comprehensive review. Journal of the American College of Surgeons 204:102–117, 2007.

Singer M. New techniques in the treatment of common perianal diseases: Stapled hemorrhoidopexy, botulinum toxin, and fibrin sealant. Surgical Clinics of North America 86: 937–967, 2006.

Chapter Self-Test Questions

Circle correct answer. After you have responded to questions, check your answers in Appendix A.

1. The term "hemorrhoid" refers to well-vascularized subcutaneous tissues that cushion the anal lining during defecation. What factor(s) predisposes to development of pathology in these structures?

   a. Repetitive straining

   b. Increased intra-abdominal pressure

   c. Infection

   d. None of the above

   e. Both a. and b.

2. How do internal hemorrhoids typically present?

   a. Bleeding

   b. Pain

   c. Prolapse

   d. Both a. and c.

3. What is the treatment for bleeding, first-degree hemorrhoids?

   a. Elastic band ligation

   b. Epinephrine injection

   c. Stool softeners

   d. None of the above

4. What is the key physical finding that is found with rectal prolapse and distinguishes this entity from prolapsing internal hemorrhoids?

   a. Concentric mucosal folds

   b. Longitudinal mucosal folds

   c. Absence of mucosal folds

   d. Ulcerations in mucosa

5. What is the most common location for an anal fissure?

   a. Anterior midline

   b. Posterior midline

   c. Lateral aspects of anal canal

See the testbank CD for more self-test questions.

HERNIAS

Louis Reines, MD, and Robert A. Kozol, MD

I. Anatomy

A. Layers of abdominal wall (from superficial to deep)

1. Skin and subcutaneous fat

2. Scarpa fascia (not real fascia)

3. External oblique

    a. Outermost layer of abdominal wall

    b. Arises from lower eight ribs and serratus anterior

    c. External oblique aponeurosis

        i. Stretches between anterosuperior iliac spine (ASIS) and pubic tubercle to form inguinal ligament

        ii. Forms external ring

        iii. Inguinal ligament reflects medially the pectin pubis to form lacunar ligament

4. Internal oblique

    a. Middle layer of abdominal wall musculature

    b. Superior border of inguinal canal

    c. Fibers run superomedially at right angles to external oblique

    d. Aponeurosis of internal oblique

        i. Contributes to anterior and posterior rectus sheath above arcuate line but only to anterior rectus sheath below it

    e. Conjoint tendon (fused fascia of internal oblique and transversalis)

        i. 5%–10% of people have true "tendon" here

5. Transversus abdominis

    a. Innermost layer of abdominal wall musculature

      b. Inferior edge of transversus abdominis aponeurosis inserts onto Cooper ligament, which is formed from periosteum and fascial condensations along posterior aspect of superior pubic ramus

   6. Transversalis fascia

   7. Properitoneal fat

   8. Peritoneum

B. Inguinal canal in three dimensions (Fig. 20.1)

   1. Deep inguinal ring

      a. Defect in transversalis fascia

      b. Halfway between ASIS and pubic tubercle

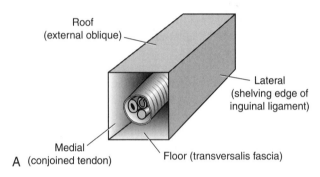

Inguinal canal

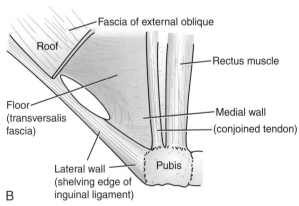

FIGURE 20.1 (A) Schematic drawing of the left inguinal canal in three dimensions as viewed from the patient's feet toward the head. (B) Anatomy of the right inguinal canal, with the "roof" (exterior oblique fascia) removed.

    c. Spermatic cord (male) and round ligament (female) exit abdominal cavity and enter inguinal canal through it
2. Inguinal canal
    a. Courses from deep inguinal ring to superficial inguinal ring
    b. Borders of inguinal canal
        i. Transversalis fascia: posterior border
        ii. External oblique fascia: anterior border
        iii. Arching fibers of transversus abdominis and internal oblique: superior border
        iv. Inguinal and lacunar ligament: inferior border
3. Hesselbach triangle
    a. Triangular region of abdominal wall through which direct hernia protrudes
        i. Inferior epigastric artery—lateral border
        ii. Rectus sheath—medial border
        iii. Inguinal ligament—inferior border
4. Spermatic cord
    a. Passes through deep inguinal ring with vas deferens, testicular vessels, and obliterated processus vaginalis
    b. Relation of abdominal wall and spermatic cord
        i. External oblique = external spermatic fascia
        ii. Internal oblique = cremaster muscle
        iii. Transversalis fascia = internal spermatic fascia
        iv. Peritoneum = processus vaginalis
5. Iliopubic tract
    a. Thickening of endoabdominal fascia
    b. Transversalis fascia and iliopsoas fascia meet (at the deepest aspect of the inguinal ligament)
    c. Courses from ASIS to pubic tubercle
6. Femoral canal
    a. Potential space for herniation deep to inguinal ligament

> The mnemonic for femoral anatomy from lateral to medial is NAVEL: femoral *n*erve, femoral *a*rtery, femoral *v*ein, empty space, *l*igament.

    b. Boundaries
        i. Femoral vein: lateral border
        ii. Inguinal ligament: superoanterior border

      iii. Lacunar ligament: posterior border

      iv. Cooper ligament: medial border

  7. Sensory-motor anatomy of inguinal canal

    a. L1 nerve root

      i. Iliohypogastric nerve

      ii. Ilioinguinal nerve—runs superior to spermatic cord through superficial ring to innervate scrotum or labia majora

    b. Genitofemoral nerve

      i. Enters inguinal canal inferior to deep inguinal ring

      ii. Motor to cremaster

      iii. Sensory to scrotum and medial thigh

C. Types of hernia (based on anatomy)

  1. Indirect inguinal hernia (Fig. 20.2)

    a. Protrusions through deep internal ring

    b. Pass laterally to inferior epigastric vessels

    c. Arise because patent processus vaginalis

    d. Sac present within cremaster muscle

    e. Located on anteromedial aspect of cord

    f. Most common abdominal wall hernia

    g. Affects males more than females

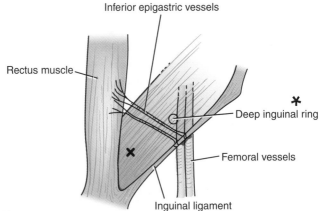

✱ Site of indirect inguinal hernia

✖ Site of direct inguinal hernia

Figure 20.2 Anatomy of the groin. X demonstrates site of direct hernias through floor of inguinal canal, medial to epigastric vessels.

2. Direct inguinal hernia (see Fig. 20.2)
   a. Arises medial to inferior epigastric vessels
   b. Occurs because of weak transversalis fascia
   c. Incarceration rare
   d. Affects males more than females
3. Femoral hernia (Fig. 20.3)
   a. Affects females more than males
   b. Common in elderly
   c. Prone to incarceration and strangulation
   d. Peritoneal outpouching through femoral canal
4. Umbilical hernia
   a. Site of weakness where urachus, round ligament, obliterated umbilical arteries converge
   b. Incarceration rare
   c. Regress spontaneously in children younger than 5 years
5. Epigastric hernia
   a. Occurs in linea alba superior to umbilicus
   b. Occurs in males more often than in females
   c. 20% multiple
6. Spigelian hernia
   a. Occurs where the transversus abdominis aponeurosis joins the edge of the rectus sheath from the semilunar line

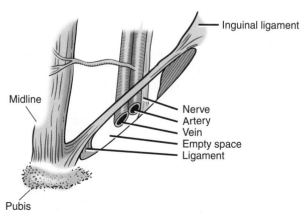

FIGURE 20.3 Anatomy of femoral vessels at the inguinal level.

   b. High likelihood of incarceration
7. Incisional hernia
   a. Develops through surgical incision in abdominal wall
   b. 0.5%–13.9% of patients undergoing abdominal surgery
   c. Risk factors
      i. Chronic obstructive pulmonary disease (COPD)
      ii. Obesity
      iii. Use of steroids
      iv. Wound infections
      v. Ascites
      vi. Male gender
      vii. Increasing age
      viii. Poor nutrition
8. Lumbar hernia
   a. Occurs in posterior abdominal wall region
   b. Sites of origin
      i. Superior lumbar triangle
      ii. Inferior lumbar triangle
9. Obturator hernia
   a. Acquired defect through obturator canal
   b. Occurs in elderly women
   c. Associated with radicular pain during abduction or internal
      rotation of knee (Howship-Romberg sign)
10. Richter hernia
   a. Less than full circumference of bowel becomes entrapped
      in an abdominal wall defect
   b. Associated with ischemia but not obstruction
11. Littre hernia
   a. Richter hernia containing Meckel diverticulum
12. Sliding hernia
   a. Part of hernia sac composed of the herniating organ

 It is important to avoid injury to viscera during repair of a sliding hernia.

II. History
   A. Asymptomatic
      1. Notice lump in groin or vaginal area
      2. Notice lump in scrotal sac

      3. Reducible: hernia contents returned to anatomic position
manually

  B. Mild symptoms

      1. Sensation of pulling or tearing

      2. Radiates to scrotum or labia majora

  C. Pain

      1. Associated with incarceration or inability to return contents of
hernia to their normal position without surgery

      2. Prolonged incarceration can lead to strangulation or compromise of blood supply to hernia contents

III. Physical Examination Supine and Standing

  A. Inspect

      1. Mass

      2. Erythema

      3. Asymmetry

  B. Palpate

      1. Bulge

      2. Mass

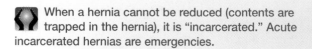

> When a hernia cannot be reduced (contents are trapped in the hernia), it is "incarcerated." Acute incarcerated hernias are emergencies.

      3. Asymmetry of cord

  C. Place fingertip into inguinal canal and have patient perform
Valsalva maneuver

      1. Indirect inguinal hernia

      2. Direct inguinal hernia

  D. Role of radiologic imaging when physical examination equivocal

      1. Ultrasound

      2. Computed tomography (CT) scan

  E. Abdominal wall defects

      1. Radiologic imaging may play greater role in diagnosis and
plan for repair than for inguinal hernias

IV. Management

  A. Observation (new data)

      1. When no hernia can be detected

      2. When patient has several comorbidities

3. When patient's life expectancy is short and hernia is asymptomatic

 Asymptomatic hernias in the elderly may be observed long-term.

B. Surgery
   1. Conventional: native tissue (non-mesh repairs)
      a. Bassini repair: sutures approximate reflection of inguinal ligament to conjoint tendon
      b. McVay repair: similar to Bassini but conjoint tendon brought to Cooper ligament

    A McVay repair also closes the femoral empty space and thus can be used to repair femoral hernias.

      c. Lichtenstein repair: tension-free repair utilizing mesh
      d. Shouldice repair: imbrication of floor of inguinal canal
      e. Plug and patch: placing plug of mesh in hernia defect and overlaying patch of mesh on inguinal floor

   Mesh repairs have replaced native tissue repairs (Bassini and McVay) for more than 90% of inguinal hernia repairs.

      f. High ligation: ligation and transection of indirect hernia sac without repair of inguinal floor (used only in children)
   2. Laparoscopic
      a. Indications
         i. Bilateral inguinal hernias
         ii. Recurring hernias
         iii. Patient preference
         iv. Need to resume full activity as soon as possible
      b. Approach to operation
         i. Placement of mesh patch over deep inguinal ring and floor of inguinal canal in preperitoneal area
         ii. Transabdominal preperitoneal approach (TAPP)
            (1) Intraperitoneal trocars

(2) Dissection of peritoneal flap and placement of mesh deep to peritoneum

(3) Must avoid "triangle of pain" (bordered by iliopubic tract and lateral aspect of spermatic vessels and contains femoral cutaneous and genitofemoral nerve) and "triangle of doom" (bordered by medial aspect of spermatic vessels and vas deferens and contains iliac vessels)

iii. Totally extraperitoneal approach (TEP)

(1) Pneumatic dilatation of preperitoneal space

(2) Mesh held in place by peritoneum

V. Outcomes

A. Table 20.1 shows some typical outcomes.

TABLE 20.1

Comparison of Open Versus Laparoscopic Mesh Repair of Inguinal Hernia

	Open Repair	Laparoscopic Repair
Use of local anesthesia	11.5%	<1%
Intraoperative complications	1.9%	4.8%
Early postoperative complications	19%	24%
Serious complications	<1%	1.1%
Recurrence rate at 2 years	4.9%	10.1%

Based on data from EU Hernia Trialists Collaboration: Laparoscopic compared with open methods of groin hernia repair: Systematic review of randomized controlled trials. British Journal of Surgery 87:860–867, 2000; and from Neumayer L, Giobbie-Harder A, Jonasson O, et al: Open mesh versus laparoscopic mesh repair of inguinal hernia. New England Journal of Medicine 350:1819–1827, 2004.

MENTOR TIPS DIGEST

- The mnemonic for femoral anatomy from lateral to medial is NAVEL: femoral *n*erve, femoral *a*rtery, femoral *v*ein, *e*mpty space, *l*igament.
- It is important to avoid injury to viscera during repair of a sliding hernia.
- When a hernia cannot be reduced (contents are trapped in the hernia), it is "incarcerated." Acute incarcerated hernias are emergencies.
- Asymptomatic hernias in the elderly may be observed long-term.
- A McVay repair also closes the femoral empty space and thus can be used to repair femoral hernias.
- Mesh repairs have replaced native tissue repairs (Bassini and McVay) for more than 90% of inguinal hernia repairs.

Resources

EU Hernia Trialists Collaboration. Laparoscopic compared with open methods of groin hernia repair: Systematic review of randomized controlled trials. British Journal of Surgery 87:860–867, 2000.

Fitzgibbons RJ. Nyhus and Condon's hernia, 5th ed. Philadelphia, Lippincott Williams & Wilkins, 2002.

Fitzgibbons RJ, et al. Watchful waiting vs repair of inguinal hernia in minimally symptomatic men: A randomized clinical trial. Journal of the American Medical Association 295:285-292, 2006.

Kozol R, Kosir M, et al. A prospective, randomized study of open vs. laparoscopic inguinal hernia repair. Archives of Surgery 132:292–295, 1997.

Neumayer L, Giobbie-Hurder A, Jonasson O, et al: Open mesh versus laparoscopic mesh repair of inguinal hernia. New England Journal of Medicine 350:1819–1827, 2004.

Chapter Self-Test Questions

Circle the correct answer. After you have responded to the questions, check your answers in Appendix A.

1. The medial aspect of the internal oblique aponeurosis joins the aponeurosis of the transversus abdominis to form the conjoined tendon in what percentage of individuals?

   a. 20%–30%

   b. 5%–10%

   c. 100%

   d. 60%–70%

2. The deep inguinal ring is a defect in which layer of the abdominal wall musculature?

   a. Internal oblique

   b. Scarpa fascia

   c. External oblique

   d. Transversalis fascia

3. Match the following abdominal wall layers to their respective spermatic cord layers:

a. External oblique	1. Processus vaginalis
b. Internal oblique	2. Internal spermatic fascia
c. Transversalis fascia	3. Cremaster muscle
d. Peritoneum	4. External spermatic fascia

4. This nerve arises from the L1 and L2 nerve roots and provides motor innervation for the cremaster muscle:

   a. Iliohypogastric

   b. Genitofemoral

   c. Ilioinguinal

   d. External spermatic

5. An elderly woman presents to the emergency room complaining of a painful bulge in her groin. She states that she has never noticed this bulge; on physical examination it is hard, painful to touch, lies below the inguinal ligament, and the overlying skin is slightly erythematous. She has been vomiting for the past several hours, and her abdomen is distended. What is the diagnosis?

a. Incarcerated direct inguinal hernia

b. Incarcerated femoral hernia

c. Necrotic inguinal lymph node

d. Incarcerated lumbar hernia

See the testbank CD for more self-test questions.

21

ANEURYSMAL DISEASE

Brian Park, MD, and James O. Menzoian, MD

I. Definition

A. *Aneurysm:* focal dilation of an artery, with at least a 50% increase in diameter compared with normal expected diameter of the artery

B. Most common type of aneurysm: abdominal aortic aneurysm (AAA)

II. Pathophysiology

A. Most common pathology: atherosclerotic degeneration
1. Focal intimal thickening
2. Reduced elastin in media and adventitia
3. Chronic inflammation with activation of proteases
4. AAA enlarges ~4 mm per year but accelerates as becomes larger (law of Laplace)
5. Multifactorial process also involving genetic factors, cigarette smoking, and aging (incompletely understood).

B. Connective tissue disorders
1. Marfan syndrome (defect in fibrillin)
2. Ehlers-Danlos syndrome (defect in collagen type III)
3. Aneurysms occur at younger ages and more diffusely

C. Infectious (mycotic aneurysms)
1. Bacterial, not fungal, origin
2. Related to tertiary syphilis

D. Other aneurysms: iliac, popliteal, femoral, visceral, renal, carotid, upper extremity

 Incidence of coexisting AAA when popliteal/lower extremity aneurysm diagnosed is 20%.

    1. Most common visceral aneurysm: splenic (higher incidence in pregnant women)

 Most common visceral aneurysm is splenic artery aneurysm.

  E. Pseudoaneurysms (false aneurysm)
    1. Caused by vascular trauma
    2. Lack all three layers of the vascular wall

III. Epidemiology

  A. Rupture of AAA is 13th most common cause of death in United States

 Mortality for ruptured AAA is 50% of those who survive to operation.

  B. 15,000 deaths annually
  C. 50% mortality if patients survive to operative repair
  D. Greater than 80% mortality overall
  E. AAA in men over age 55: 4.3%
  F. AAA in women over age 55: 2.1%
  G. More common in men (5:1)
  H. 100,000 new cases per year
  I. Incidence increases with aging
  J. Whites:African American (3.5:1)

IV. Prevention

  A. Major risk factors for AAA
    1. Smoking (most important)
    2. Age
    3. White
    4. Hypercholesterolemia
    5. Genetic: 10%–20% incidence in families
    6. Coronary artery and peripheral vascular disease
    7. Chronic obstructive pulmonary disease (COPD)
  B. Modification of risk factors
    1. Medical management of hypertension
    2. Smoking cessation

Most important risk factor for AAA is smoking.

   3. Lipid-modifying strategies (diet, exercise, pharmacologic agents: statins)
C. Screening
   1. Who
      a. Males older than age 65 with history of smoking
      b. Males and females with family history of AAA
   2. How
      a. Routine history and physical examination
      b. Abdominal x-ray—"eggshell calcifications" not reliable finding
      c. Abdominal ultrasound (US)
      d. Confirm via computed tomography angiogram (CTA) or magnetic resonance angiogram (MRA)

V. Signs and Symptoms
A. Asymptomatic
   1. Most common presentation
   2. Assess risk factors and focus physical examination
B. Back and abdominal pain
   1. Nonspecific
   2. Spinal erosion can cause back pain
C. Embolization
   1. Ischemia in lower extremities from AAA thrombus: 5% incidence
D. Dissection: disruption of intima and media of aneurysms (rare)
E. Acute rupture: 12% of initial presentation for AAA
F. Greater the diameter, greater risk of rupture
   1. 4–4.9 cm:1%/yr
   2. 5–5.9 cm: 10%/yr
   3. 6 cm: 20%/yr
   4. 7 cm: 30%/yr

VI. History and Physical Examination
A. Symptoms of back pain, early satiety, lower extremity ischemia
B. Assess risk factors present: hypertension, smoking, diet
C. Physical examination

1. Hypertension
2. Abdominal bruits
3. Pulsatile midline abdominal mass
4. Aorta may be more prominent in very thin individuals

 Most common clinical presentation of AAA is asymptomatic/incidental finding.

VII. Differential Diagnosis
   A. Intra-abdominal mass
   B. Other visceral aneurysm

VIII. Management
   A. Medical management of risk factors
     1. Control of hypertension
     2. Smoking cessation
     3. Lipid-lowering diet, exercise, drugs
   B. Appropriate diagnostic studies: initially US, followed by CTA or MRA
   C. Surgical intervention
     1. Open repair with prosthetic graft (Fig 21.1)
       a. Through anterior midline or retroperitoneal approach
       b. Distal and proximal cross-clamping synthetic graft with/without iliac limbs
       c. Close aneurysm sac over graft to prevent aortoenteric fistula (highly lethal late complication)
       d. Operative mortality 4%–5%

 Most common complication following AAA repair is myocardial infarction.

     2. Endovascular aneurysm repair (EVAR) (Fig. 21.2)
       a. Access bilateral femoral arteries
       b. Deploy endograft below renal arteries (proximal fixation) and to iliac (distal fixation) under fluoroscopic guidance
       c. Operative mortality 1%–3%
     3. Ruptured AAA—50% die in the field, 50% of those reaching hospital die

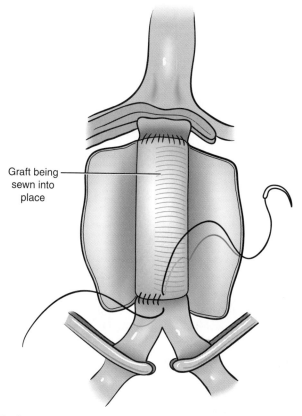

Graft being sewn into place

FIGURE 21.1 Open repair of aneurysm with prosthetic graft. *(From Vascular Web. Provided by the Society for Vascular Surgery.)*

IX. Follow-Up

A. Surveillance CTA for EVAR every 6 months to assess for technical problems

B. Ongoing risk factor modification

C. Late rupture risk after open repair ~ 0%, EVAR 1%–3%/yr

D. Secondary intervention open repair 0%, EVAR 8.7%

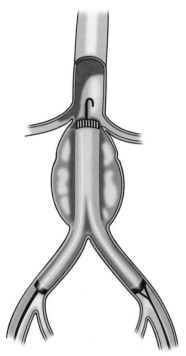

Figure 21.2 Endovascular aneurysm repair (EVAR). *(From VascularWeb Provided by the Society for Vascular Surgery.)*

 MENTOR TIPS DIGEST

- Incidence of coexisting AAA when popliteal/lower extremity aneurysm diagnosed is 20%.
- Most common visceral aneurysm is splenic artery aneurysm.
- Mortality for ruptured AAA is 50% of those who survive to operation.
- Most important risk factor for AAA is smoking.
- Most common clinical presentation of AAA is asymptomatic/incidental finding.
- Most common complication following AAA repair is myocardial infarction.

Resources

Eliason JL, Clouse WD. Current management of infrarenal abdominal aortic aneurysms. Surgical Clinics of North America 87, 2007.

Townsend CM. Sabiston textbook of surgery, 18th ed. Philadelphia, Elsevier, 2007.

Chapter Self-Test Questions

Circle the correct answer. After you have responded to the questions, check your answers in Appendix A.

1. What is the most common cause of death following open AAA repair?

   a. Stroke

   b. Graft infection

   c. Myocardial infarction

   d. Internal hemorrhage from lumbar arteries

2. What event most commonly leads to discovery of AAA?

   a. Back pain

   b. Acute rupture

   c. Embolization to extremities

   d. Diagnosis on CTA scan for unrelated disease

3. Which of the following is not an indication for repair of AAA?

   a. Symptomatic aneurysm

   b. Aneurysm greater than 5 cm

   c. Rapidly expanding AAA

   d. Family history of AAA rupture

4. Which of the following is the best initial diagnostic modality for AAA?

   a. Abdominal x-ray

   b. Abdominal CTA scan

   c. Abdominal US

   d. Abdominal MRA

5. Which of the following is true regarding infected aortic grafts?

   a. Graft infections may be adequately treated with broad spectrum antibiotics

   b. Graft infections may be adequately treated with specific, targeted antibiotics

   c. Infected grafts must be excised, and a new graft must be sewn in place

   d. Infected grafts must be excised, and an extra-anatomic bypass is required

See the testbank CD for more self-test questions.

22

PERIPHERAL VASCULAR OCCLUSIVE DISEASE

Brian Park, MD, and James O. Menzoian, MD

I. Definition

A. Peripheral vascular occlusive disease (PVOD) is partial or complete occlusion of a peripheral artery caused by atherosclerosis.

II. Pathophysiology

A. Most common disorder: atherosclerotic degeneration
  1. Focal intimal thickening
  2. Reduced elastin in media and adventitia
  3. Chronic inflammation with activation of proteases
  4. Vascular smooth muscle cells: abnormal proliferation in response to injury
  5. Multifactorial process involving genetic factors and aging (incompletely understood)

B. Most common sites: arterial branching (related to sheer stress)
  1. Infrarenal aorta
  2. Iliofemoral arteries (especially superficial femoral artery)
  3. Carotid bifurcation
  4. Popliteal arteries

C. Acute thromboembolism
  1. Tolerance of acute ischemia varies by end organ
    a. Brain: 4–8 minutes
    b. Heart: 17–20 minutes
    c. Lower extremity: 6 hours
  2. Embolism
    a. Cardiac origin 80% of cases

Cardiac events are the most common source of acute embolic debris.

b. Emboli from rheumatic valvular disease
c. Bacterial or fungal emboli: risk with intravenous (IV) drug abuse
d. Aortic plaque emboli
e. Cryptogenic (unknown source) 10%–15% cases
3. Reperfusion syndrome
   a. Revascularization of acutely ischemic limbs
   b. Release of toxins from cells: myoglobin, lactic acid, potassium
   c. Edema can lead to compartment syndrome
   d. Oxygen-derived free radicals injure tissue
4. Clinical presentation: 5 P's (pain, pallor, pulselessness, paralysis, poikilothermy)
5. Management
   a. Medical emergency
   b. Prompt anticoagulation with heparin
   c. Thrombolytic therapy by intra-arterial infusion (if limb viable and there is time)
   d. Urgent surgical intervention in severely threatened limb
   e. Evaluation for the source
   f. In situ thrombosis of diseased vessel or embolus
   g. Consideration for compartment syndrome and fasciotomy
D. Other arteriopathies
   1. Thromboangiitis obliterans (Buerger disease)
      a. Related to heavy cigarette smoking
      b. Rest pain, gangrene, ulceration
      c. Remission with smoking cessation

 In Buerger disease, remission occurs with smoking cessation.

   2. Takayasu arteritis (pulseless disease)
      a. Common in younger females (Asian and eastern European)
      b. Disease of aorta and major branches
      c. Cerebral ischemia
      d. Upper extremity claudication

3. Giant cell (temporal) arteritis
   a. Patients older than 50 years; 2:1 female predominance
   b. Affects temporal, vertebral, aortic branches
   c. Retinal artery involvement can lead to blindness

 Temporal arteritis requires prompt steroids to prevent blindness.

   d. Requires prompt steroid treatment
4. Raynaud phenomenon
   a. Recurrent vasospasm of digits
   b. Related to cold exposure or stress
   c. Treatment: avoid cold, calcium channel blockers

III. Epidemiology
   A. Affects 25 million persons in United States
   B. Many individuals may be asymptomatic; estimated that 2 million Americans have symptomatic disease reducing quality of life
   C. Prevalence increases with age in men and women
      1. 5% before age 50 years
      2. 10% by age 65 years
      3. Over 25% by age 80 years
   D. No difference in overall prevalence by gender
   E. Symptomatic PVOD more prevalent in men

IV. Prevention
   A. Major risk factors
      1. Smoking (most important)
      2. Diabetes
      3. Hypertension
      4. Hypercholesterolemia
      5. Obesity
      6. Age
      7. Male gender
      8. Genetic: 10%–20% incidence in families
   B. Modification of risk factors
      1. Medical management of hypertension, diabetes, obesity
      2. Smoking cessation
      3. Lipid-modifying strategies (diet; exercise; pharmacologic agents, e.g., statins)

C. Screening
  1. Routine history and physical examination
  2. Noninvasive studies
    a. Ankle-brachial index (ABI)/segmental limb pressures (ankle blood pressure/arm blood pressure): gives accurate assessment of limb perfusion and is reliable measure of PVOD: ABI <7 = claudication; <4 = rest pain or tissue loss
    b. Pulse volume recording (PVR): volumetric measurement of blood flow at various levels of the extremity, especially helpful in diabetic patients who have calcified blood vessels resulting in an artificially elevated ABI
    c. Exercise testing ABI/PVR in the presence of a significant arterial stenosis/obstruction exercise will reduce ABI
    d. Duplex ultrasonography
    e. Confirm with computed tomography angiogram (CTA)/magnetic resonance angiogram (MRA)

V. Signs and Symptoms

A. Intermittent claudication
  1. Reproducible muscle pain with exercise
  2. Relieved by rest
  3. Pain occurs one level below lesion (buttock pain for aortoiliac lesions, calf pain with superficial femoral artery (SFA) lesions, etc.)
B. Rest pain
  1. Foot or toe pain while supine
  2. Improves with dependency/ambulation
C. Tissue loss
  1. Ischemic ulcers
  2. Gangrene
D. Acute embolism
  1. White, painful, cold limb
E. Leriche syndrome: buttock claudication, diminished femoral pulses, impotence (aortoiliac disease)

VI. History and Physical Examination

A. Symptoms of claudication, rest pain, tissue loss, embolism
B. Assess presence of risk factors: smoking, diabetes, lipids, hypertension

C. Physical examination
1. Complete peripheral pulse examination
   a. Femoral, popliteal, posterior tibial, dorsalis pedis
2. Hair loss
3. Shiny, thin skin
4. Thickened toenails
5. Peripheral bruits
6. Foot/leg ulcers
7. Assess cardiac rhythm

VII. Differential Diagnosis
A. Neurogenic limb pain: spinal stenosis
B. Popliteal artery entrapment syndromes (usually young people)
C. Exertional compartment syndrome (usually young athletic individuals)
D. Arthritis
E. Diabetic neurogenic foot ulcer/infection

VIII. Management
A. Medical management of risk factors
1. Smoking cessation

 Most important modifiable risk factor for PVOD is smoking.

2. Lipid-lowering diet, exercise, drugs
3. Good diabetic control
4. Control of hypertension
5. Obesity treatment
6. Antiplatelet agents: aspirin, dipyrimadole, clopidogrel
7. Appropriate diagnostic studies: ABI/PVR, duplex ultrasound, angiography as needed for treatment
B. Surgical intervention
1. Open bypass with vein or prosthetic graft
   a. All bypasses require inflow, outflow, conduit
   b. Saphenous vein is superior conduit choice: 90%

 In lower extremity bypass graft with saphenous vein, typically there is 90% patency at 1 year.

c. Prosthetic grafts have higher failure and infection rates
d. Prosthetic graft infection requires excision
e. Cardiac events are greatest source of perioperative mortality

 Cardiac events are the greatest source of mortality following lower extremity revascularization procedures.

f. 5-year patient survival rate after femoral-popliteal bypass: 50%

C. Angioplasty with or without stenting
  1. Good results for iliofemoral disease: 85% patency at 1 year

 In aortoiliac angioplasty with stenting, typically there is 85% patency at 1 year.

  2. Stents not used below popliteal artery (break with motion)
  3. Angioplasty below iliofemoral level: 50% patency at 1 year

IX. Follow-Up

A. Routine follow-up visits every 6 months to assess for recurrent symptoms
B. Surveillance by noninvasive studies
C. Ongoing risk factor modification
D. Risk of limb loss following bypass: 10% over 10 years
E. Nondiabetic patients with lower extremity ischemia: 70% survival at 5 years

 MENTOR TIPS DIGEST

- Cardiac events are the most common source of acute embolic debris.
- In Buerger disease, remission occurs with smoking cessation.
- Temporal arteritis requires prompt steroids to prevent blindness.
- Most important modifiable risk factor for PVOD is smoking.
- In lower extremity bypass graft with saphenous vein, typically there is 90% patency at 1 year.
- Cardiac events are the greatest source of mortality following lower extremity revascularization procedures.

- In aortoiliac angioplasty with stenting, typically there is 85% patency at 1 year.

Resources

Aquino R. Natural history of claudication: Long-term serial follow-up study of 1244 claudicants. Journal of Vascular Surgery 34:962–970, 2001.

Imparato AM. Intermittent claudication: Its natural course. Surgery 78:795–799, 1975.

Sontheimwer DL. Peripheral vascular disease: Diagnosis and treatment. American Family Physician 73, 2006.

Chapter Self-Test Questions

Circle the correct answer. After you have responded to the questions, check your answers in Appendix A.

1. Tolerance of acute ischemia varies by end organ. What are some approximate times?

    a. brain: _____–_____ minutes

    b. heart: _____–_____ minutes

    c. lower extremity: _____ hours

2. Clinical presentation of acute thromboembolism typically involves the 5 P's, which are:

    P_____

    P_____

    P_____

    P_____

    P_____

3. List the signs and symptoms that constitute Leriche syndrome:

_____

_____

_____

See the testbank CD for more self-test questions.

23

CHAPTER

CEREBROVASCULAR DISEASE

Brian Park, MD, and James O. Menzoian, MD

I. Pathophysiology
   A. Underlying disorder: atherosclerosis of cerebral vasculature
      1. Most common location: carotid bifurcation
      2. Other locations: vertebral arteries (lead to cerebellar symptoms), aortic arch, innominate artery
   B. Basic mechanisms of strokes
      1. Embolization atherosclerotic plaques (most common)
      2. Thrombotic occlusion
      3. Hypoperfusion (drop in cardiac output with reduction in cerebral perfusion)
   C. Stroke: hypoperfusion to cerebral or cerebellar cortex leading to infarction
      1. Types of strokes:
         a. Ischemic: atherothrombotic, thromboembolic, lacunar
         b. Hemorrhagic: intracerebral, subarachnoid
         c. Completed
         d. Stroke-in-evolution (progressive worsening of neurologic deficit)
         e. Transient ischemic attacks (TIA) (symptoms resolve in 24 hours)

II. Epidemiology
   A. Strokes are third most common cause of death in United States

 Strokes are the third most common cause of death in the United States.

259

B. New strokes 160/100,000 population per year

C. 750, 000 stroke per year

D. 200,000 fatal strokes per year

E. Two-thirds of survivors are permanently disabled

F. Health-care cost $10 billion per year

III. Prevention

    A. Major risk factors for strokes

        1. Hypertension (most important)

        2. Extracranial vascular atherosclerosis (carotid artery bifurcation)

        3. Intracranial vascular atherosclerosis

        4. Smoking

        5. Hypercholesterolemia

        6. Cardiac disease (atrial fibrillation, myocardial infarction, mitral stenosis, infective myocarditis, left ventricular hypertrophy)

        7. Diabetes

        8. Obesity

    B. Modification of risk factors

        1. Medical management of hypertension (40% reduction in strokes with good hypertension management)

        2. Smoking cessation

        3. Lipid-modifying strategies (diet, exercise, pharmacologic agents: statins)

        4. Anticoagulation for atrial fibrillation

    C. Screening

        1. Surveillance duplex ultrasound (US)

        2. Magnetic resonance angiogram (MRA)/computed tomography angiogram (CTA) to confirm lesions

IV. Signs and Symptoms

    A. Stroke

        1. Dominant hemisphere symptoms: left

            a. Motor dysfunction right face or hand.

            b. Loss of vision left eye

            c. Sensory symptoms of right body (numbness, paresthesias)

            d. Aphasias

        2. Nondominant hemisphere symptoms: right

            a. Similar symptoms on contralateral distribution

            b. No aphasias (speech centers on left)

B. Transient ischemic attacks
   1. Temporary neurologic deficit lasting less than 24 hours
   2. Usually resolve in 15 minutes

 In TIA, stroke symptoms resolve in 24 hours.

C. Amaurosis fugax
   1. Monocular blindness in one eye that is reversible
   2. Described as "shade being pulled down"
D. Vertebrobasilar symptoms (cerebellar)
   1. Motor dysfunction (weakness, paralysis, not lateralizing)
   2. Sensory dysfunction (numbness, paresthesias, not lateralizing)
   3. Loss of vision, both eyes
   4. Loss of balance, vertigo symptoms

V. History and Physical Examination
A. Symptoms of amaurosis fugax, transient ischemic attacks, strokes by history
B. Assess risk factors: hypertension, smoking, diet, diabetes, coronary heart disease
C. Physical examination
   1. Hypertension
   2. Cardiac rhythm
   3. Carotid bruits: unreliable with high-grade lesions
   4. Retinal hemorrhages, Hollenhorst plaques on ophthalmoscope examination

VI. Differential Diagnosis
A. Brain tumor
B. Syncope
C. Migraine
D. Seizures
E. Vestibulopathy
F. Neurologic disorder: amyotrophic lateral sclerosis, multiple sclerosis, transient global amnesia
G. Psychosomatic origin: conversion disorders
H. Malingering

VII. Management
A. Medical management of risk factors
1. Control of hypertension
2. Smoking cessation
3. Lipid-lowering diet, exercise, drugs (statins)
4. Aspirin and clopidogrel (Plavix) may reduce risk of stroke

B. Surgical intervention for extracranial carotid artery disease
1. Carotid endarterectomy: gold standard (Fig. 23.1)
   a. Removal of diseased intima, media, plaque

 Structures of carotid arteries removed during endarterectomy are intima, media, and plaque.

   b. Closure of artery with patch (synthetic or xenograft)
   c. Absolute risk reduction of stroke confirmed through major trials (North American Symptomatic Carotid Endarterectomy Trial, Asymptomatic Carotid Atherosclerosis Study, European Carotid Surgery Trial): symptomatic carotid disease 17%/2 years; asymptomatic carotid disease 53%/5 years

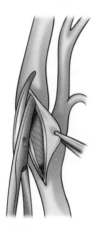 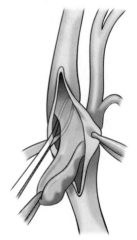

FIGURE 23.1 Carotid endarterectomy. *(From VascularWeb. Provided by the Society for Vascular Surgery.)*

2. Carotid angioplasty with stenting (Fig. 23.2)

   a. Angioplasty to dilate stenosed carotid arteries

   b. Stenting to maintain patency and stabilize plaque

   c. Neuroprotection to prevent embolization during procedure

VIII. Follow-Up

A. Routine follow-up visits every 6 months to assess for recurrent symptoms

B. Surveillance duplex US to assess vessel patency

C. Ongoing risk factor modification

D. Restenosis rate 10% in first year

 Rate of restenosis of carotid arteries after repair is 10% at 1 year.

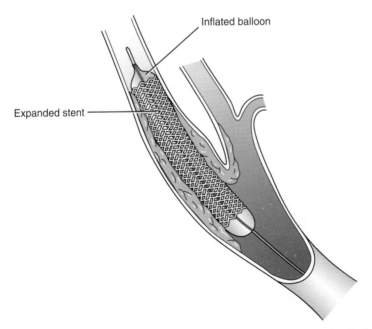

FIGURE 23.2 **Carotid angioplasty with stenting.** *(From VascularWeb. Provided by the Society for Vascular Surgery.)*

E. Recurrent carotid stenosis within 2 years: caused by myointimal hyperplasia

 Cause of recurrent stenosis within 2 years is myointimal hyperplasia.

F. Recurrent stenosis beyond 2 years: caused by progression atherosclerosis

 Cause of recurrent stenosis 2 or more years after repair is progression of atherosclerosis.

 MENTOR TIPS DIGEST

- Strokes are the third most common cause of death in the United States.
- In TIA, stroke symptoms resolve in 24 hours.
- Structures of carotid arteries removed during endarterectomy are intima, media, and plaque.
- Rate of restenosis of carotid arteries after repair is 10% at 1 year.
- Cause of recurrent stenosis within 2 years is myointimal hyperplasia.
- Cause of recurrent stenosis 2 or more years after repair is progression of atherosclerosis.

Resources

Park B, Aiello F, Dahn M, et al. Follow-up results of carotid angioplasty with stenting as assessed by duplex ultrasound surveillance. American Journal of Surgery 192:583–588, 2006.

Park B, Mavanur A, Dahn M et al. Clinical outcomes and cost comparison of carotid artery angioplasty with stenting versus carotid endarterectomy. Journal of Vascular Surgery 44:270–276, 2006.

van der Vaart MG. Endarterectomy or carotid artery stenting: The quest continues. American Journal of Surgery 195: 259–269, 2008.

Chapter Self-Test Questions

Circle the correct answer. After you have responded to the questions, check your answers in Appendix A.

1. The most common cause of cerebral ischemia (stroke) is:

   a. Cerebral hypoperfusion from hypotension

   b. Thrombosis and occlusion of the carotid artery

   c. Embolization of carotid plaques

   d. Embolization from cardiac thrombus

2. A patient presents to your office with an asymptomatic cervical bruit. Which is the most appropriate course of action?

   a. Work up the patient with a CTA

   b. Work up the patient with an MRA

   c. Work up the patient with a carotid duplex US

   d. Schedule the patient for carotid endarterectomy

3. Which of the following is true regarding carotid endarterectomy?

   a. A relative risk reduction of subsequent stroke has been demonstrated for symptomatic patients

   b. An absolute risk reduction of subsequent stroke has been demonstrated for asymptomatic patients

   c. Endarterectomy involves excision of the intima, media, plaque, and tunica

   d. Carotid endarterectomy must always be performed with a patch material

4. Embolization of plaque debris to which artery is responsible for amaurosis fugax?

   a. Temporal artery

   b. Facial artery

   c. Optic artery

   d. Retinal artery

5. Which of the following is true regarding cerebrovascular disease?

   a. The most common complication following carotid reconstruction is stroke

   b. Aphasias commonly occur with right-side strokes

   c. Carotid endarterectomy requires general anesthesia

   d. The most common cause of carotid restenosis in the perioperative period is technical error

See the testbank CD for more self-test questions.

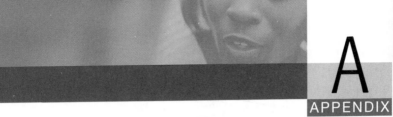

ANSWERS TO SELF-TEST QUESTIONS

Below are the answers to the self-test questions that appear at the end of most chapters.

Part I: The Basics

Chapter 1: Introduction to the Surgical Service

1. Identify the film (e.g., "This is a CT scan of the abdomen")
2. Be calm
3. Be systematic
4. Do not jump to the obvious finding as you may miss something (again, be systematic)

2. *A*dmit to
   *D*iagnosis
   *C*ondition
   *V*itals
   *A*llergies
   *A*ctivity
   *N*ursing orders
   *D*iet
   I's and O's
   *M*eds
   *I*V fluids
   *L*abs

3. Use mnemonics; visualize the patient from head to toe and cover all body systems.

Chapter 3: Fluids and Electrolytes

1. 1500
2. 136
3. Hypocalcemia
4. HCO_3^-

Chapter 4: Surgical Nutrition

1. Males = 66 + (13.7 × weight in kg) + (5 × height in cm) −
(6.8 × age in yr)
Females = 65.6 + (9.6 × weight in kg) + (1.7 × height in cm) −
(4.7 × age in yr)
2.
    a. 16–40
    b. 200–360
    c. 3.5–5.5
3. Early enteral nutrition reduces postoperative mortality; prevents intestinal mucosal atrophy; supports gut-associated immunologic shield; attenuates hypermetabolic response to injury; less expensive than parenteral nutrition; fewer complications than parenteral nutrition

Chapter 5: Minimally Invasive Surgery

1.
    a. Solubility
    b. Lack of flammability
2. Hypercarbia (usually transient); myocardial suppression; may induce arrhythmias; embolism (rare given high solubility of CO_2); respiratory effects (decreased lung compliance [>30%]; decreased functional residual capacity; need for hyperventilation to excrete an increased CO_2 load)
3. acidosis; arrhythmias; subcutaneous emphysema; pneumothorax; pneumomediastinum; atelectasis; gas embolism

Part II: Emergencies

Chapter 6: Shock

1. d. Systemic vascular resistance (SVR) × cardiac output (CO)
Response: HR × SV = CO; CO/BSA = cardiac index (CI), SV/BSA = stroke volume index (SVI)

2. c. Bacteremia
Response: SIRS is a type of vasodilatory shock that occurs without evidence of infection. Septic shock is vasodilatory shock as a result of infection.

3. b. Inadequate tissue perfusion
Response: Whereas hypotension, tachycardia, and acidosis may be present during many shock states, inadequate tissue perfusion is a uniting feature of all types of shock.

4. c. 3:1
Response: It has been empirically observed that approximately 300 mL of crystalloid is required to compensate for each 100 mL of blood loss. This 3:1 rule is a good beginning point for fluid resuscitation but is obviously not a hard-and-fast rule for those with massive hemorrhage.

5. d. Pneumonia
Response: Cardiogenic shock is characterized by a decreased pumping ability of the heart, which leads to inadequate tissue perfusion. It most commonly occurs in association with, and as a direct result of, acute myocardial infarction. Pneumonia may cause septic shock, but it is not usually a cause cardiogenic shock.

Chapter 7: Trauma Evaluation and Resuscitation

1. c. Grade III shock, 30%–40% blood volume loss
2. a. Homicide
3. Lateral cervical spine, chest, pelvis

Chapter 8: Burns

1. b. 18%
Response: The Rule of Nines is for adults. Children's percentages are different.

2. c. Narrow-spectrum antibacterial
Response: Silver sulfadiazine (Silvadene) is generally the initial topical medication for burns. It is a broad-spectrum antibacterial.

3. d. UO>30 mL/hr

Chapter 9: Gastrointestinal Hemorrhage

1. Diverticulosis
2. No treatment required (bleeding usually stops spontaneously)
3. Occult; massive
4. Colonoscopic snare cautery polypectomy

Part III: Core Topics

Chapter 10: Breast

1. Fibroadenoma
2. Core-needle biopsy
3. Age; inherited genetic mutations (*BRCA-1* or *BRCA-2*); personal or family history of breast cancer; personal or family history of ovarian cancer; biopsy-proven atypical hyperplasia; high breast density; reproductive factors (early menarche, late menopause, nulliparity); long-term use of hormone replacement therapy

Chapter 11: Thyroid and Parathyroids

1. Permanent voice change (RLN injury) (3%); neck hematoma requiring reoperation (1%); permanent hypoparathyroidism (severe hypocalcemia) (5%–8%)
2. Recurrent laryngeal nerves (left and right)
3. Lobectomy plus isthmusectomy

Chapter 12: Acute Abdomen and Appendicitis

1. d. All of the above
2. c. B-HCG
3. a. Mesenteric ischemia
4. b. 7%
5. c. Early zoster before vesicles erupt

Chapter 13: Stomach and Duodenum

1. d. Left gastroepiploic artery
Response: The left gastric artery, splenic artery, and common hepatic artery are the three main divisions of the celiac trunk. The left gastroepiploic artery is a branch of the splenic artery.

2. b. *Helicobacter pylori*
Response: *H. pylori* is a helical-shaped gram-negative microaerophilic acidophilic bacterium that infects various areas of the stomach and duodenum. Many cases of peptic ulcers, gastritis, duodenitis, and perhaps some cancers are caused by *H. pylori* infection.

3. b. They may be found in MEN type II patients
Response: A gastrinoma is a tumor that secretes gastrin. It is frequently the source of the gastrin in Zollinger-Ellison syndrome. It is most commonly found in the pancreas and duodenum. A very small percent (0.1%–1%) of patients with peptic ulcer disease have a gastrinoma. The diarrhea that results can be halted by aspiration of gastric secretions. The gastrinoma is associated with MEN type I (pancreatic tumors, parathyroid hyperplasia, and pituitary adenomas), neither MEN type IIA (medullary thyroid carcinoma, pheochromocytoma, and parathyroid hyperplasia) nor MEN type IIB (medullary thyroid carcinoma, pheochromocytoma, and mucosal neuromas).

4. a. Gastroduodenal artery
Response: The gastroduodenal artery can be the source of a significant gastrointestinal bleed, which may arise as a complication of peptic ulcer disease. The artery arises from the common hepatic artery and terminates in a bifurcation, where it splits into the right gastroepiploic artery and the anterior superior pancreaticoduodenal artery. It supplies blood to the pylorus (distal part of the stomach) and the proximal part of the duodenum.

5. c. *H. pylori* infection associated with peptic ulcer disease
Response: A perforated peptic ulcer is a surgical emergency and requires surgical repair of the perforation. Most bleeding ulcers require endoscopy urgently to stop bleeding with cautery or injection. However, a bleeding ulcer unresponsive to medical therapy requires emergency surgery. Gastric outlet obstruction and peptic ulcer disease refractory to medical treatment are the other indications for surgical treatment, although these occur less frequently. This is mainly due to the eradication of *H. pylori* infection and the use of proton pump inhibitor therapy. The presence of *H. pylori* infection is not an indication for surgical management of a peptic ulcer.

Chapter 14: Hepatobiliary System

1. a. Hepatic vein
Response: The portal triad consists of the portal vein, hepatic artery, and bile duct.

2. d. Surgery and albendazole
Response: Percutaneous drainage of echinococcal abscess is not recommended because spillage of cyst can cause severe anaphylactic reaction. Antiparasite therapy, albendazole, or mebendazole is given 1 month before surgical drainage and is continued postoperatively to reduce recurrence.

3. b. Hepatic hemangioma
Response: Hepatic hemangioma is the most common benign liver tumor. Focal nodular hyperplasia is the second most common. Benign liver tumor is more common in females.

4. b. Cholate and chenodeoxycholate
Response: Cholate and chenodeoxycholate are primary bile salts. They are deconjugated to secondary bile salts; deoxycholate and lithocholate by gut bacteria.

5. b. Cholangitis
Response: The patient presents with sepsis: hypotension and altered mental status. He presents with Reynold pentad (fever, RUQ pain, jaundice, hypotension, altered mental status). The history suggests cholangitis. The most likely cause of cholangitis is obstruction resulting from choledocholithiasis. However, not all patients with choledocholithiasis end up with cholangitis. Patients with necrotizing gallstone pancreatitis can present similarly but with elevated lipase. This patient will require emergency ERCP for decompression of the biliary system.

Chapter 15: Spleen

1. c. Splenic hilum
Response: An accessory spleen ("supernumerary spleen," "splenule," or "splenunculus") is a small nodule of splenic tissue found in some people in the area of the spleen, most commonly in the splenic hilum. Accessory spleens may be isolated or connected to the spleen by thin bands of splenic tissue. They vary in size from that of a pea to that of a plum.

2. a. Coronary ligament
Rsponse: The coronary ligament of the liver refers to parts of the peritoneal reflections that hold the liver to the inferior surface of the diaphragm. The gastrosplenic, splenorenal, and phrenocolic ligaments are the peritoneal ligaments that support the spleen.

3. d. Sickle cell disease
Response: Sickle cell disease is a relatively rare indication for splenectomy. Trauma, hypersplenism, hereditary spherocytosis, and ITP are much more common indications for splenectomy.

4. b. *S. aureus*
Response: Because splenectomy causes an increased risk of overwhelming sepsis due to encapsulated organisms (such as *S. pneumoniae* and *H. influenzae*), the patient should be immunized, if possible, prior to removal of the spleen. Vaccination for pneumococcus, *H. influenzae,* and meningococcus should be given preoperatively if possible.
5. b. The pediatric population
Response: Asplenic individuals are at increased risk of postsplenectomy sepsis, a fulminant and rapidly fatal illness that complicates bacteremic infections due to encapsulated pathogens. The incidence of this syndrome is highest in children who undergo splenectomy in infancy.

Chapter 16: Pancreas

1. c. Inferior pancreaticoduodenal artery, which is a branch off the superior mesenteric artery
Response: The inferior pancreaticoduodenal artery (a branch off the superior mesenteric artery) and the superior pancreaticoduodenal artery (a branch off the gastroduodenal artery) supply the pancreas.
2. d. Ethanol and gallstones
Response: There are many known causes of acute pancreatitis; however, ethanol and gallstones are the two most common causes of acute pancreatitis in the United States.
3. b. Bruising of the flank
Response: Grey Turner sign refers to bruising of the flanks. This sign takes 24–48 hours to appear and predicts a severe attack of acute pancreatitis, with mortality rising from 8%–10% to 40%. It may be accompanied by Cullen sign (blue-black bruising of the area around the umbilicus). George Grey Turner was a British surgeon.
4. a. Broad-spectrum antibiotics
Response: Broad-spectrum antibiotics are not used in the initial treatment of acute pancreatitis. If necrotizing pancreatitis is diagnosed, antibiotics may be indicated, but this remains a topic of controversy.
5. b. Amylase
Response: Amylase is not part of Ranson criteria. Ranson criteria, which were introduced in 1974, are a clinical prediction rule for predicting the severity of acute pancreatitis.

Chapter 17: Small Bowel

1. 2% of population; 2% become symptomatic; present within the first 2 years of life; 2 types of mucosa (ileal and ectopic); 2 feet from the ileocecal valve; 2 cm in size
2. Crohn disease; celiac sprue; immunosuppression; transplant; systemic chemotherapy; SLE; AIDS
3. Erythema nodosum; erythema multiforme; pyoderma gangrenosum

Chapter 18: Colon

1. **d.** Both a. and c.
2. **b.** 1.5 m
3. **a.** Splenic flexure
4. **b.** N-butyrate
5. **d.** Anaerobes

Chapter 19: Anorectum

1. **e.** Both a. and b.
2. **d.** Both a. and c.
3. **c.** Stool softeners
4. **a.** Concentric mucosal folds
5. **b.** Posterior midline

Chapter 20: Hernias

1. **b.** 5%–10%
2. **d.** Transversalis fascia
3. **a-4, b-3, c-2, d-1**
4. **b.** Genitofemoral
5. **b.** Incarcerated femoral hernia

Chapter 21: Aneurysmal Disease

1. **c.** Myocardial infarction
2. **d.** Diagnosis on CTA scan for unrelated disease
3. **d.** Family history of AAA rupture
4. **c.** Abdominal US
5. **d.** Infected grafts must be excised, and an extra-anatomic bypass is required

Chapter 22: Peripheral Vascular Occlusive Disease

1.
- **a.** 4–8
- **b.** 17–20
- **c.** 6

2. Pain, pallor, pulselessness, paralysis, poikilothermy

3. Buttock claudication, diminished femoral pulses, impotence

Chapter 23: Cerebrovascular Disease

1. c. Embolization of carotid plaques

2. c. Work up the patient with a carotid duplex US

3. b. An absolute risk reduction of subsequent stroke has been demonstrated for asymptomatic patients

4. d. Retinal artery

5. d. The most common cause of carotid restenosis in the perioperative period is technical error

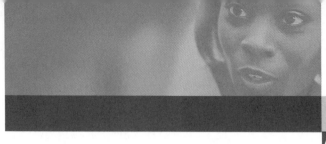

ABBREVIATIONS

Abbreviation	Complete Term
5-ASA	5-aminosalicylic acid (mesalazine)
5-HIAA	5-hydroxyindoleacetic acid (serotonin metabolite)
6-MP	6-mercaptopurine
AAA	abdominal aortic aneurysm
ABCDE, etc.	airway, breathing, circulation, disability, exposure, etc. (priorities in emergency situations)
ABI	Ankle-Brachial Index
ACE	Angiotensin-converting enzyme
AFP	alpha-fetoprotein
AIDS	acquired immunodeficiency syndrome
AIS	Abbreviated Injury Scale
ALT	alanine transaminase
AMI	acute myocardial infarction
AMPLE	allergies, medications, past illnesses/pregnancy, last meal, events/environment
APR	abdominoperineal resection
ARDS	acute respiratory distress syndrome
ARF	acute renal failure
AS	aortic stenosis
ASCA	anti-*Saccharomyces cerevisiae* antibodies
ASIS	anterior superior iliac spine
AST	aspartate transaminase
ATP	adenosine triphosphate
AV	arteriovenous
AXR	abdominal x-ray
B-HCG	beta–human chorionic gonadotropin
BCC	basal cell carcinoma
BE	barium enema
BM	bowel movement
BMI	Body Mass Index
BRBPR	bright red blood per rectum

BSA	body surface area
BUN	blood urea nitrogen
ca	carcinoma
CA 19-9	carbohydrate antigen 19-9
CBC	complete blood count
CCK	cholecystokinin
CEA	carcinoembryonic antigen; carotid endarterectomy
CHF	congestive heart failure
CO	carbon monoxide; cardiac output
CO_2	carbon dioxide
COPD	chronic obstructive pulmonary disease
CRF	chronic renal failure
CT	computed tomography
CTA	computed tomographic angiography
CV	cardiovascular
CVP	central venous pressure
CXR	chest x-ray
DCIS	ductal carcinoma in situ
DI	diabetes insipidus
DIC	disseminated intravascular coagulation
DM	diabetes mellitus
DNA	deoxyribonucleic acid
DPL	diagnostic peritoneal lavage
ECF	extracellular fluid
ECG/EKG	electrocardiogram
ECHO	echocardiogram
ECV	extracellular volume
ED	emergency department
EGD	esophagogastroduodenoscopy
EH	external hemorrhoids
ERCP	endoscopic retrograde cholangiopancreatography
ETT	endotracheal tube
EUA	examination under anesthesia
EVAR	endovascular aneurysm repair
FAMMM	familial atypical multiple mole melanoma (syndrome)
FAP	familial adenomatous polyposis
FAST	focused assessment with sonography for trauma
FENa	fractional excretion of sodium
FNH	focal nodular hyperplasia
FOBT	fecal occult blood test
GB	gallbladder

GCS	Glasgow Coma Scale
GDA	gastroduodenal artery
GERD	gastroesophageal reflux disease
GGT	gamma-glutamyl transferase
GI	gastrointestinal
GIST	gastrointestinal stromal tumor
GYN	gynecologic
HALS	hand-assisted laparoscopic surgery
HCC	hepatocellular carcinoma
HEENT	head, eyes, ears, nose, throat
IH	internal hemorrhoid
HIDA scan	hepatobiliary iminodiacetic acid scan
HIV	human immunodeficiency virus
HNPCC	hereditary nonpolyposis colorectal cancer
HP	*Helicobacter pylori*
HPT	hyperparathyroidism
HPV	human papillomavirus
HR	heart rate
HUS	hemolytic-uremic syndrome
IC	ileocecal
ICF	intracellular fluid
ICU	intensive care unit
ICV	intracellular volume
IF	interstitial fluid
IMA	inferior mesenteric artery
INR	International Normalized Ratio
IS	incentive spirometry
ISS	Injury Severity Score
ITP	idiopathic thrombocytopenic purpura
IV	intravenous
IVC	inferior vena cava
IVF	intravenous fluid
JP	Jackson-Pratt (drain)
LARP	left/anterior, right/posterior (vagus nerves)
LBO	large-bowel obstruction
LCIS	lobular carcinoma in situ
LDH	lactate dehydrogenase
LFTs	liver function tests
LGI	lower gastrointestinal
LLQ	left lower quadrant (abdomen)
LN	lymph node
LR	lactated Ringer (solution)

LT	ligament of Treitz
LUQ	left upper quadrant (abdomen)
MD	Meckel diverticulum
MEN	multiple endocrine neoplasia
MI	myocardial infarction
MPD	myeloproliferative disorder
MRA	magnetic resonance angiography
MRCP	magnetic resonance cholangiopancreatography
MRI	magnetic resonance imaging
MSOF	multiple systems organ failure
NAVEL	nerve, artery, vein, empty space, ligament (femoral anatomy)
NG	nasogastric
NGT	nasogastric tube
NPO	nothing by mouth *(nil per os)*
NS	normal saline
NSAID	nonsteroidal anti-inflammatory drug
OCP	oral contraceptive pill
OR	operating room
PACU	post-anesthesia care unit
pANCA	perinuclear antineutrophil cytoplasmic antibodies
PDS	polydioxanone suture
PID	pelvic inflammatory disease
PO/p.o.	by mouth *(per os)*
PPH	procedure for prolapse and hemorrhoids
PPI	proton pump inhibitor
PQRST	palliative or provocative factor, quality, radiation, severity, temporal sequence (mnemonic for interviewing patients with pain)
PRBCs	packed red blood cells
PSS	postsplenectomy sepsis
PT	prothrombin time
PTC	percutaneous transhepatic cholangiography
PTH	parathyroid hormone
PTHrp	parathyroid hormone–related peptide
PTX	pneumothorax
PUD	peptic ulcer disease
PVOD	peripheral vascular occlusive disease
PVR	pulse volume recording
RBCs	red blood cells
RLL	right lower lobe (lung)
RLN	recurrent laryngeal nerve

RLQ	right lower quadrant (abdomen)
RR	respiratory rate
RTS	Revised Trauma Score
RUQ	right upper quadrant (abdomen)
SB	small bowel
SBO	small-bowel obstruction
SBP	systolic blood pressure
SCC	squamous cell carcinoma
SCD	sequential compression device
SFA	superficial femoral artery
SIADH	syndrome of inappropriate antidiuretic hormone
SIRS	systemic inflammatory response syndrome
SLE	systemic lupus erythematosus
SMA	superior mesenteric artery
SMV	superior mesenteric vein
SOB	shortness of breath
SV	stroke volume
SVR	systemic vascular resistance
TAPP	transabdominal preperitoneal
TBSA	total body surface area
TBW	total body water
TEM	transanal endoscopic microsurgery
TEP	totally extraperitoneal
TIA	transient ischemic attack
TIPS	transjugular intrahepatic portosystemic shunt
TME	total mesorectal excision
TNF	tumor necrosis factor
TNM	tumor, nodes, metastasis
TPN	total parenteral nutrition
TRISS	Trauma Injury Severity Score
TURP	transurethral resection of the prostate
UC	ulcerative colitis
UGI	upper gastrointestinal
UO	urine output
US	ultrasonography
WBCs	white blood cells

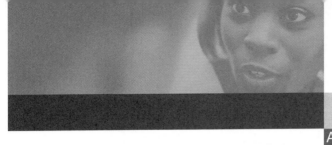

KEY CONTACTS AND NOTES

Physician Contacts

NAME	CONTACT
Dr	Home phone:
	Mobile phone:
	Pager:
	Other:
Dr	Home phone:
	Mobile phone:
	Pager:
	Other:
Dr	Home phone:
	Mobile phone:
	Pager:
	Other:

Community Resources and Phone Numbers

NAME/PROGRAM	PHONE NUMBERS
Sexual and Physical Abuse	
Substance Abuse	
Communicable Diseases (HIV, Hepatitis, Others)	
Homeless Shelters	
Child/Adolescent Hotlines	
Suicide Hotlines	
Hospitals (General, Veterans, Psychiatric)	
Medicare	
Medicaid	
Other	

Facility Phone Numbers

NAME/PROGRAM	PHONE NUMBERS
Main	Phone:
	Fax:
Laboratory	Phone:
	Fax:
Radiology	Phone:
	Fax:
Physical Therapy	Phone:
	Fax:
ECG/EEG	Phone:
	Fax:
Outpatient Scheduling	Phone:
	Fax:
Emergency	Phone:
	Fax:
Operating Suite	Phone:
	Fax:
Admissions	Phone:
	Fax:
Billing	Phone:
	Fax:
Medical Records	Phone:
	Fax:
Medical Staff Office	Phone:
	Fax:
Other important numbers	Phone:
	Fax:

Formulary Notes Specific to Your Facility

Other Important Information

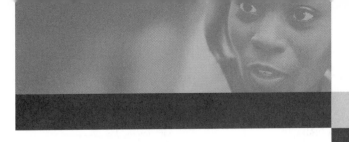

INDEX

Entries followed by *f* or *t* denote figures and tables, respectively.